FAMILY
HEALTH
MATTERS

Tai Chi
for beginners
and the 24 Forms

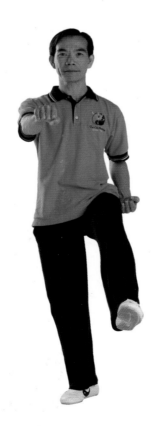

The authors and anyone involved in the production and distribution of this book will not be held responsible in any way whatsoever for any injury or consequence that may arise as a result of following the instructions given in this book. Readers who engage in these activities do so at their own risk.

Limelight Press Pty Ltd
Unit 15, 6 Thames Street
Balmain NSW 2041
ABN 80 095 617 897

Published by Limelight Press Pty Ltd 2006   Second Printing 2009

National Library of Australia
Cataloguing-in-Publication data:

Lam, Paul.
Tai chi for beginners and the 24 forms.

Bibliography.
Includes index.
ISBN 0 9775361 1 4.

1. Tai chi. 2. Health. I. Title. (Series : Family health matters).

613.7148

Photographs copyright Dr Paul Lam

Designed by Lena Lowe

Printed in Korea through Four Colour Imports, LTD. Louisville, Kentucky

Tai Chi
for beginners
and the 24 Forms

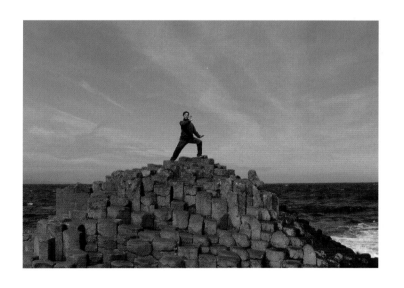

DR PAUL LAM   NANCY KAYE

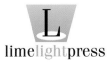

limelightpress

Contents

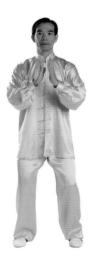

Foreword

One could call us "The Odd Couple". He's Australian–Chinese; she's American. He lives in Sydney; she lives in California. He's a number (maths) person; she's a word (language) person. What made us get together to write a book? Our common dedication to tai chi and our determination to share the love of the art with others.

We could say that this book and its contents were all our idea. In a way, that's true. But it's the numerous tai chi beginners and enthusiasts we've talked to who have shown us the way. They've helped us decide what this book should be and what should be included. For example, they wanted a book that was easy and enjoyable to read. They wanted it to teach them authentic tai chi through simple instructions that work. Rather than learn tai chi as a martial art, they preferred to focus on the health benefits. Lastly, they wanted a reference book.

We've tried to offer beginners all of the above and more. In *Tai Chi for Beginners and the 24 Forms*, we've made a conscientious effort to help the reader build a solid foundation right from the start, as well as giving him or her a taste of higher level tai chi. And perhaps most important, we've done our best to make tai chi fun to learn.

Our main goal with this book is to get you, the reader, "hooked" on tai chi so that the art will become part of your life. We couldn't wish you anything more beneficial, fulfilling—or enjoyable.

Dr Paul Lam and Nancy Kaye

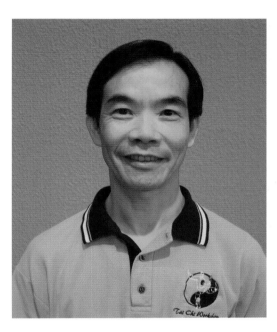 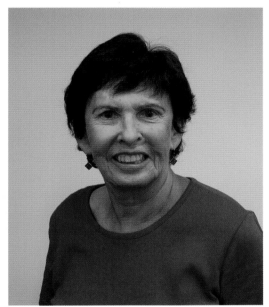

How to use this book

First and foremost, you should know that we have organized this book by layers, just the way you, as beginners, would progress. We have given you three steps or stages: beginning, intermediate and ideas for progress. And that's the way we all learn best, in progressive steps. You'll find, for example, that in Chapter 4, we add to your understanding of things you learned in Chapter 3.

From experience, we've learned that teaching step by step enables beginners to gain the necessary knowledge and skill in the easiest and most effective way.

If knowing the background of tai chi is very important to you, you can read through all the chapters first (especially Part 2). But if you lean more towards "doing" rather than reading, you can simply read the introductions to Chapters 1 and 2 and then go straight into the exercises in Chapter 3. Later on, you can go back to more in-depth reading.

As a tai chi beginner and beyond, you can use this book by itself or in conjunction with classes and/or the instructional DVDs *Tai Chi for Beginners* and *The 24 Forms*. If you don't have an instructor, please be sure to make adjustments according to your own ability and requirements, and follow the instructions carefully. In Chapter 3, there's a suggested lesson plan with detailed instructions for each step.

For tai chi instructors

The book is useful as a reference for advanced practitioners as well as tai chi instructors. Instructors can use Dr Lam's *Six Easy Steps* for classes without applying for permission to do so. However, be aware that it is your responsibility to teach safely. We provide a guide to safe practice in Chapter 2.

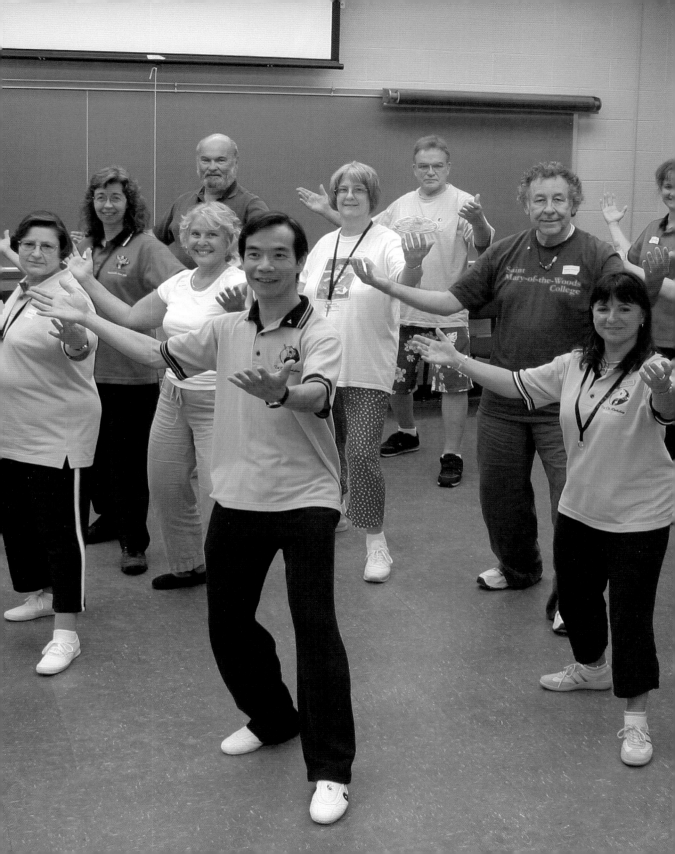

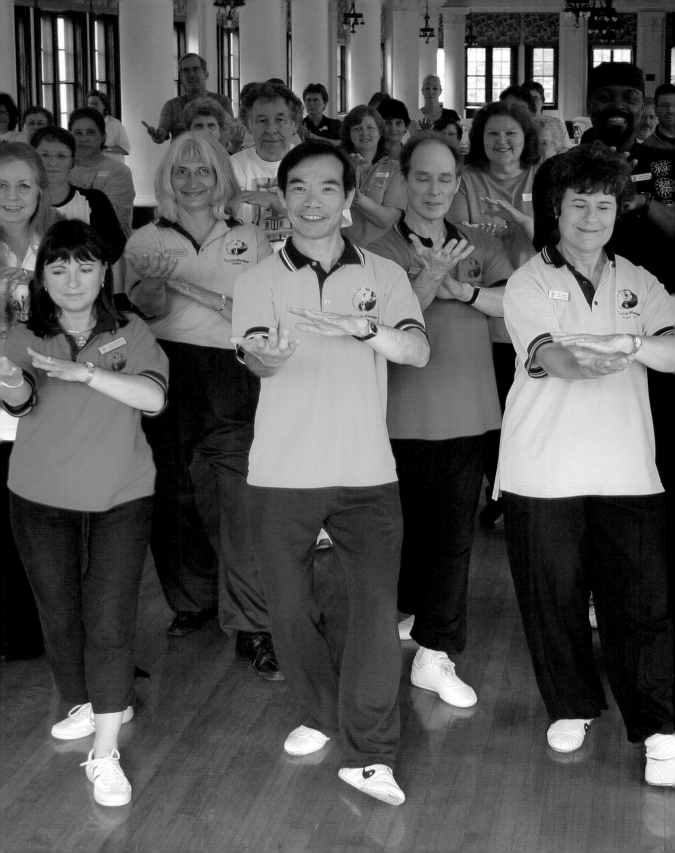

PART 1

FOR THE BEGINNER

CHAPTER 1

WHAT CAN TAI CHI DO FOR YOU?

T ai chi, although a martial art, is practised primarily for its health benefits. And for good reasons. Scientific studies show that it helps chronic conditions such as arthritis, heart disease and diabetes, and that it also improves balance, prevents falls and reduces stress.

The practice of tai chi includes cultivating *qi*, the vital life energy, which, in turn, relaxes us and uplifts our spirits. Most importantly, tai chi is an enjoyable form of exercise that people of any age can learn and practise.

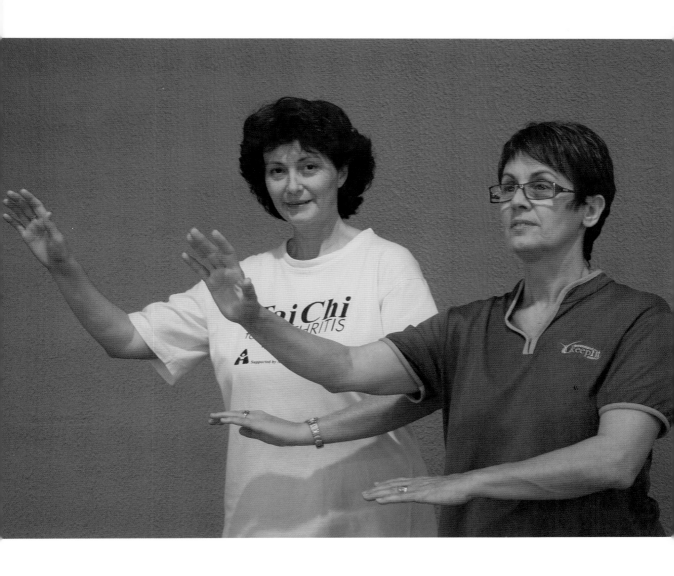

In a nutshell, tai chi can keep you healthy and happy. It's remarkably effective for relaxation, health and fitness. Besides that, it's fun.

Studies have shown that tai chi works magic on health, improving conditions such as arthritis, heart disease, diabetes, respiratory diseases and other chronic illnesses. In addition, it improves balance, prevents falls, aids good posture, and helps build immunity to disease. And if that's not enough, tai chi also counters mental illness, depression and stress.

Almost anyone can learn tai chi. Learning is inexpensive; tai chi can be practised almost anywhere. For the most part, the movements are slow and gentle, and you can easily adjust the degree of exertion to suit yourself. So …

Just what is tai chi?

Originating in ancient China, tai chi is an effective exercise for health of mind and body. Although an art with great depth of knowledge and skill, it can be easy to learn and soon delivers its health benefits. For many, it continues as a lifetime journey.

There are many styles and forms of tai chi, the major ones being Chen, Yang, Wu, another Wu (actually two different words in Chinese) and Sun. Each style has its own unique features, although most styles share similar essential principles. These include the mind being integrated with the body; fluidity of movement; control of breathing; and mental concentration. The central focus is to enable the qi, or life force, to flow smoothly and powerfully throughout the body. Total harmony of the inner and outer self comes from the integration of mind and body, achieved through the ongoing practice of tai chi.

Here's to your health

Medical and fitness authorities stress that effective exercise for health should include three components: cardiovascular fitness, muscular strength and flexibility.

Cardiovascular fitness

Cardiovascular fitness means better heart–lung capacity. A good supply of blood and oxygen is essential for maintaining your health and for healing any disease.

In 1996, a study was carried out involving 126 post-heart-attack patients. They were randomly assigned to participate in either a tai chi class or an aerobic exercise class or a non-exercise support group. The patients from the tai chi group came out with better cardiovascular fitness and lower blood pressure than patients from the non-exercise group. Furthermore, 80 per cent of the people in the tai chi group continued

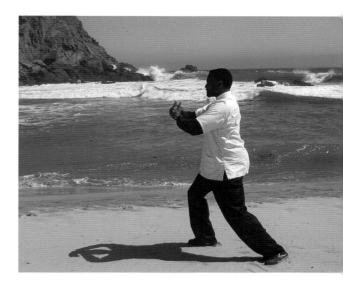

the practice of tai chi while the non-exercise support group retained only 10 per cent of its original membership. The aerobic group retained fewer of its members than the tai chi group and their diastolic blood pressure did not improve.

THE YIN, THE YANG AND THE QI

Tai chi is based on traditional Chinese medicine, *qigong* (the method of cultivation of qi) and martial art. Traditional Chinese medicine is based on a holistic understanding of humans as part of the universe and their constant interaction with the elements in the universe.

The ancient Chinese believed that all things in nature were composed of *yin* and *yang*. While yin and yang are two polar opposites, they're entirely complementary. Yin is viewed as softer, more pliant, yielding, feminine and sometimes negative, while yang appears more masculine, harder, more rigid and more positive. In nature, everything moves towards a natural state of harmony and so yin and yang are always in total balance. Complementing each other, yin and yang form a perfect whole.

Traditional Chinese medicine emphasizes that humans should exist in natural balance with nature in a spiritual and physical sense. When we are well balanced within ourselves and in balance with nature, then we will have strong qi and be healthy.

While some of these concepts may sound a little esoteric, the concepts of yin and yang and of tai chi have been validated. Over recent years, many studies have proven tai chi's significant effect in improving many aspects of health.

The ancient Chinese regarded qi as the most important energy within the body. Qi in nature is the energy in the universe, and qi within the body is the driving power that maintains health and spirit. Everyone is born with qi, and it diminishes with age or disease. The most important feature of tai chi is that it is designed to enhance the qi effectively. And the stronger your qi, the healthier you are.

Strengthening

By strengthening our muscles, we keep our joints stable and protected. Of course, we need our muscles to move and when we move, the muscles pump fluid and blood throughout the body, improving the functions not only of the organs and joints but also the entire body.

Many well-known sports heroes suffer from osteoarthritis resulting from injuries. Yet, they are able to perform at their peak level because their strong muscles protect their joints and reduce the pain of osteoarthritis. After they retire from active sports, however, and their training lapses, their muscles weaken. Arthritis flares up. Perhaps we can conclude that had they taken up tai chi upon retirement they would have stayed in shape and enjoyed a healthier, happier retirement.

Flexibility

Flexibility improves our range of motion, making us more functional. Being flexible keeps our joints, muscles—our entire body—healthy, and allows us to be more active. Jim, a 56-year-old retired fireman, is a good example of how tai chi can improve flexibility. As a result of an on-the-job injury, Jim couldn't lift his arms any higher than his shoulders. Otherwise healthy, he experienced ongoing frustration. He couldn't reach up

to cupboards; he couldn't paint his house; he couldn't even reach a book on a shelf above his head. Jim had given up hope of ever returning to normal. Then, simply to get exercise, he took up tai chi. Within six months, normal flexibility had returned to his shoulder joints. He could reach up. His life changed.

Let's get it straight

In addition to these three main components of healthy exercise, tai chi also improves posture, an important component of health. Developing correct posture will result in less wear and tear of the joint muscles. When your posture is upright, the lung space is larger. Try taking a deep breath and expanding your chest. You'll notice that there's more space in the chest. Now try to hunch. The space in your chest diminishes, doesn't it? As you can see, the body works better in an upright posture.

Shirley suffered from lower back pain and sciatica problems for some time before she started doing tai chi. Tai chi really helped her. "I think part of the reason I got better was that tai chi strengthened my back muscles and made me conscious of keeping good posture throughout the day," she says. "I don't slouch any more. It has really made a difference."

FALLS PREVENTION

Two recent studies have confirmed the effectiveness of tai chi in reducing the likelihood of falls in older adults. The first was published by *Journal of Advanced Nursing* in 2005*. Says co-author Professor Rhayun Song (who is also a master trainer of the Tai Chi for Arthritis program): "As people get older they are more likely to experience falls and this can lead to some very serious health issues ... Our study shows that low-intensity exercise such as tai chi has great potential for health promotion as it can help older people to avoid falls by developing their balance, muscle strength and confidence."

A group of 68 older adults was divided into a tai chi group and a control group. After following the Tai Chi for Arthritis program designed by Dr Lam and based on Sun style, the tai chi group reported improved muscle strength and less risk of falls than the control group. It was concluded that the tai chi program can improve physical strength and reduce fall risk in fall-prone older adults in residential care facilities.

The second study, conducted by Sydney Central Area Health Promotion Unit between 2001 and 2004 involved approximately 700 people and was the largest fall prevention study in the world. After 16 weeks of doing a tai chi program (80 per cent of the participants did the Tai Chi for Arthritis program), the results showed that "tai chi significantly reduced the number of falls by almost 35 per cent. Tai chi also significantly reduced the risk of multiple falls by approximately 70 per cent." The study concludes: "Compared with other falls prevention interventions, the trial showed that tai chi is one of the most effective ways of preventing falls in older people".**

* Choi, J.H., Moon, J.S., and Song, R., "The Effects of Sun-style tai chi exercise on physical fitness and fall prevention in fall-prone adults", *Journal of Advanced Nursing*, 2005.

** Sydney South West Area Health Service, *Falls Prevention Newsletter*, Spring 2005.

Good posture in turn promotes better balance, thus preventing falls and the resulting injuries. Shirley goes on to say, "Tai chi has also strengthened my ankles. I was twisting and spraining them once or twice a year. Now, between my stronger ankles and better posture, I enjoy better balance, and as I get older, I'll be less likely to fall."

It's all in your head

The mind is the most important aspect of health. It's a universally accepted fact that the mind controls the body. Surely you've heard of people overcoming disabilities thanks to their positive attitude and strong mind. And tai chi, as one of the most powerful mind–body exercises, teaches the student to be aware of the intrinsic energy from which he or she can derive greater self-control and empowerment.

Almost everyone who practises tai chi recognizes its powerful effect on relaxation and concentration. Take Joanne, for example. About 10 years ago while driving, she was injured in a car accident. She suffered seven pinched nerves between her skull and her coccyx. Her frequent business travel didn't help. For years she lived in pain.

Finally, a chiropractor suggested she try tai chi. "A six-week introductory course was enough to get me hooked," says Joanne. "I found that, even in that short time, what we were doing was enough to help me start to relax, and that meant my back was finally getting a chance to heal."

Stress

You don't have to have sustained an injury to benefit from tai-chi-produced relaxation. Tai chi simply offers a tool to help you cope with busy, modern-day life by appreciating the tranquillity and nature around you.

Going hand in hand with relaxation is the alleviation of stress. As a high-energy businessperson, Joanne has truly benefited from her eight years of tai chi. "Physically, I can handle stress a lot better than I used to. I'm now aware much earlier when I'm responding to stress and can react

TAI CHI FOR ARTHRITIS

Dr Paul Lam developed the Tai Chi for Arthritis program to improve quality of life for people with arthritis. A recent study* looked at how the program affected pain, stiffness and physical functions (ability to do daily tasks) in older women with osteoarthritis. After 12 weeks, when compared to the control group, the tai chi group had 35 per cent less pain, 29 per cent less stiffness and 29 per cent more ability to perform daily tasks. They also had improved abdominal muscles and better balance.

* Song, R., Lee, E.-O., Lam, P., Bae, S.-C., "Effects of tai chi exercise on osteoarthritis", *Journal of Rheumatology*, September 2003.

appropriately. That means I don't end up with tight shoulders and headaches.

"Mentally, I find that overall I handle people and stressful situations differently. I'm more inclined to sit back, listen and evaluate a situation than I used to be," she continues. "I make much more use of energy and try to be sensitive to other people's energy to assess their state of mind and body. That's tremendously helpful in dealing with difficult people and situations."

Spirit

In the context of tai chi, the term "spirit" refers simply to the way you feel rather than any religious or occult notion. It's what you're referring to when you say, "Hey, today I'm in good spirits", or "Today I'm happy".

It's usually not easy to control your mood or spirit with your conscious mind. If it were easy, depression wouldn't be so common, nor would it be so hard for doctors to treat. The spirit or mood is largely controlled by the subconscious mind, which has an immense power over us. For instance, often you know you're depressed, but although you dislike the condition, you can't seem to get out of this mental state.

The daily stress, negativity and destructive emotions accumulate to dampen our spirit, whereas when we're close to nature, for example, or involved in a cultural activity, our psychic energy gets in balance. All too often, fast-paced Western society tips the balance to the negative side. In fact, in Western society more than 50 per cent of diseases presented to doctors are caused by mind-related problems such as stress.

Tai chi can help. The ancient Chinese were aware of the immense power of the mind or spirit. Tai chi aims to achieve harmony with nature and a balance between mental serenity and physical strength. Having better balance calms the unconscious mind.

Enhancing the qi—the vital life energy within us—during tai chi practice is the path to uplifting the spirit. Our minds can learn to enhance qi, which in turn, connects with the unconscious mind to enhance our mental attitude. Qi grows when the person is well balanced and in harmony. Once your body is relaxed and calm, and your mind receptive, your qi will begin to circulate. And that will start your spirits soaring.

CHAPTER 2

GETTING READY

Why do you want to learn tai chi?

Maybe it's for your health—physical, mental, or both. Whatever your reason, before you start on your journey of learning, define your goal. That way, you won't be just doing tai chi, you'll have something definite to work towards.

Be sure to check with your health professional before you start, as well as later if you develop any problem. We strongly recommend that you read this whole chapter before continuing on to the next.

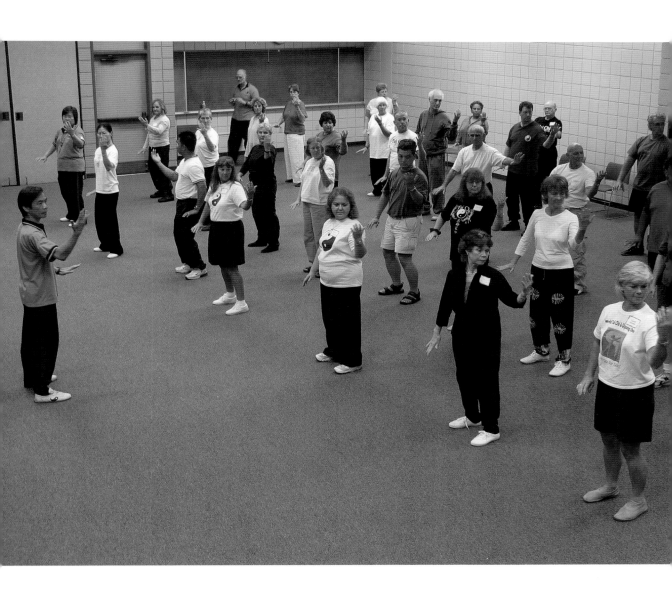

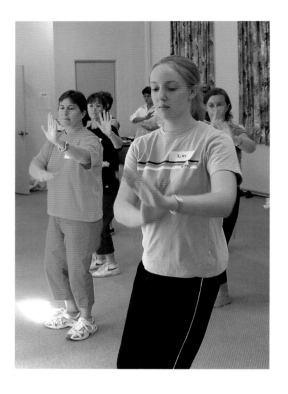

Think about your reasons for starting tai chi and what you want to achieve. Look over the checklist below and see if any of the reasons listed apply to you.

I want to do tai chi:
* to improve my health and fitness
* to alleviate stress
* to increase my flexibility and my muscle strength
* to improve my posture
* to improve existing medical conditions (arthritis, diabetes, back pain etc.)
* to improve my flow of qi
* to improve my balance
* to improve my mental health

If you decide to do tai chi and do it on a consistent basis, you'll find improvement in most, if not all, of the above.

Perhaps though, you're one of those people who have considered doing tai chi simply because you're curious. You wonder how it feels. Or maybe you've seen it done and it looks like fun. All the better. Not only are you undertaking the art with a good attitude but you just might end up with a side benefit—better health.

On the other hand, let's say since tai chi is a martial art, your long-term goal is to be a Bruce Lee. You want to learn how to fight and protect yourself. In this event,

you'd probably be better off looking into an *external* martial art, such as kung fu (as it is commonly known in the Western world) or karate. For tai chi is an *internal* martial art, meaning that it places more emphasis on internal power, the qi (life energy) and the mind. Although tai chi is one of the most effective martial arts, it will generally take a longer time to apply it to self-defence than it will with an external martial art.

Tai chi places more emphasis on improving your mental ability and health rather than your muscle power. It stresses working from within first, which helps build a strong, yet soft, inner power. This can be done no matter what your age.

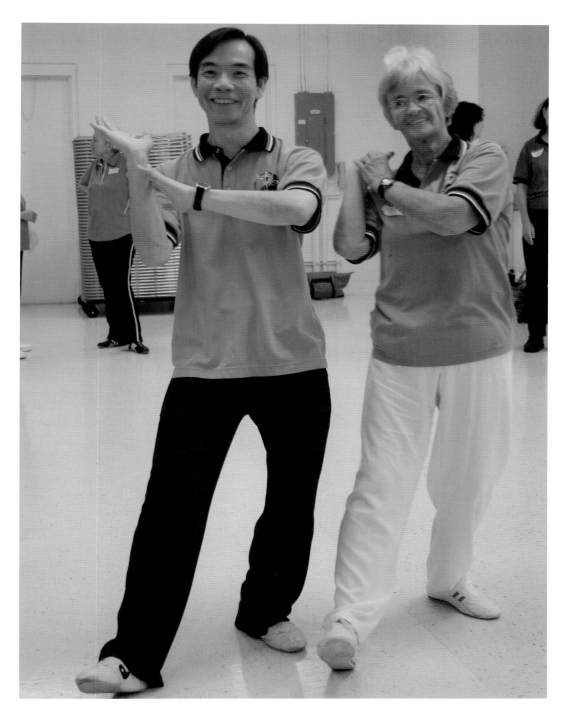

Helping tai chi achieve your goal

If you've decided to give tai chi a try, you should realize that just doing tai chi won't do much for you. To reach your goal, you'll need to form a partnership with tai chi. The formula for this is:

motivation + tai chi = success

Regular and correct practice is the major contributor to the success of learning tai chi. Be prepared to practise regularly, starting with a daily session that is realistic for you—even just a few minutes—then building up to 30–60 minutes a day. To prevent injury, warm up before each practice session and do the cool-down exercises after each session.

As you practise, listen to your body. You should feel comfortable, not over-tired and never in pain. Wear loose, comfortable clothing and flat shoes. Dress in layers, so you can easily adjust your temperature when you get too hot or too cold. Be patient. As a tai chi novice, don't expect immediate satisfaction. It takes a while for tai chi to prove its powers.

Some important practice tips

* Set a regular practice time, so your tai chi practice becomes part of your daily routine.
* When you start your practice, work out a goal for the session—for example, to remember the sequence; or a technical point, such as better control of your movements. Be sure to set a goal that is challenging but not over-challenging. Check the goal frequently as you practise. This will help you to be more focused and be in the flow.
* Set yourself a realistic deadline for achieving your goals. For example, if your goal is to lower your blood pressure, allow 12 weeks. Many studies show measurable health effects take this period of time. Meanwhile, along the way, you'll not only enjoy yourself but you'll feel better as well.
* Try to practise with someone else, especially when you're feeling unmotivated.
* Be gentle with yourself. Stay within your comfort range for level of exertion and length of practice session.

* Do all movements slowly, continuously and smoothly. As you become more familiar with the movements, they will start to flow more easily and feel more graceful.

* Breathe slowly, naturally and easily. As you become used to doing the moves, try to coordinate them with your breathing, as instructed. Return to your natural breathing if you feel any discomfort.

* Gradually build up the length and number of practice sessions, aiming for about 30–60 minutes for most days. A simple indication of how long your practice sessions should be is to make them about the same length of time as you can walk comfortably at a steady pace.

* Continue your session only for as long as you feel comfortable. Listen to your body and rest when you start to feel tired, are in pain or lose concentration.

TAKING CARE

■ If your knees become tired, stiff or painful in the bent position, stand up between movements. As your muscles become stronger, you will be able to stay comfortably in the squatting position for longer.

■ Avoid practising in a place that is too hot, too cold or windy.

■ After practising, avoid subjecting yourself to an extreme change of temperature. For example, don't immediately go from a very hot practice environment to an air-conditioned area. And when you're hot from practising, don't drink cold or chilled drinks. Subjecting the body to sudden and extreme temperature change can cause harm, a fact well known in Chinese traditional medicine and now also recognized by Western medicine.

■ Practise in an area that is clear of obstacles and has a non-slip surface with no loose mats or rugs.

■ Don't practise when you're very hungry, immediately after a big meal or when you're very upset.

■ Don't continue doing any movement that is painful or causes you discomfort. If you experience chest pains, shortness of breath, or dizziness or if additional pain in your joints persists, stop and consult your health professional.

PRECAUTIONS FOR SPECIFIC CONDITIONS

If you have any medical conditions, be sure to check with your health professional that it is okay to practise tai chi, and let your tai chi instructors know about your conditions. Below are some of the precautions you should take for specific conditions.

◼ Arthritis of the knee joints

Many people suffer from arthritis of the knee joints. Tai chi requires bent knees and maintaining the same height throughout the set of forms. This can place stress on the joints, especially of beginners. While one of the goals of tai chi is to keep the knees bent at the same height, you should work up to that very slowly (over months and even years). Stand up between movements to avoid excess stress to the knees.

◼ After a hip replacement

If you have had a hip replacement, you should avoid moving your foot across the midline. During the replacement surgery, the nerves responsible for the opposite side of the body could have been cut, thus affecting your ability to feel the position of your body. This, in turn, could affect your balance if your foot crosses the midline. Be sure to check with your doctor as to what you should and shouldn't do.

◼ Diabetes and hypoglycaemia

One of the significant dangers for people with diabetes who undertake exercise is hypoglycaemia, or low blood glucose. When the blood glucose gets too low, loss of consciousness and even brain damage can result. Hypoglycaemia affects you if you have diabetes and are being treated with medications or injections.

Exercise causes a high consumption of energy and therefore blood glucose can be depleted rapidly. The body has an efficient system to regulate blood glucose so that it stays in the right range. However, as medication or injectable insulin aims to lower blood glucose, it may interfere with the body's regulatory system and cause hypoglycaemia. This is why you should let your doctor know what kind of exercise you're doing, and heed the doctor's advice and precautions. For care of hypoglycaemia, you can obtain information from your local diabetes foundation or from their website.

Dress the part

What should you wear to practise tai chi? The key word here is comfort. Wear loose, comfortable clothes and flat shoes. For everyday practice, clothing made of cotton is ideal because it allows your skin to breathe and absorbs sweat. Stretchy clothing, such as a lycra leotard, allows for free movement, but it isn't good for tai chi since it sticks closely to the skin and thus inhibits the flow of qi (which travels along meridians, or energy channels, that are close to the surface of the skin). For the same reason, avoid tight elastic around your waist or ankles, because, again, this might restrict the flow of qi.

In winter, consider dressing in layers. You might be cold when you start practising, but once you work up a sweat you might want to remove some layers.

Summer presents a similar situation. Layers are necessary in case you get too hot, but also in case a sudden wind comes up or the temperature drops and you then need to put some clothes back on.

Footwear

Some people like to practise tai chi in bare feet, but we don't recommend it. Shoes give you good support and help your balance. Furthermore, the ground may be uneven or dirty. Also, if your feet get cold, it could impede the flow of qi. (If, however, you really like practising tai chi in bare feet, remember to find an even, clean surface with a suitable temperature.)

The ideal practice shoes should:
* feel comfortable and soft
* be lightweight
* have broad-base support in the soles to help you balance
* have shock-absorbent pads in the soles to minimize injury

Lace-up shoes such as the martial art shoes made by Adidas or New Balance are suitable, although they're not designed specifically for tai chi practitioners; thus, they may not offer good base support or shock absorbency. Traditional Chinese-made, flat-bottom cloth shoes are good for most tai chi styles. Recently, China has also developed a martial art shoe with a broadened base; these shoes vary in quality, however, so take care to choose good ones.

Don't worry if you don't feel better immediately. Give yourself time for tai chi to work its magic.

Ready … set … go!

You've set your goal. You've read the practice instructions. You've even outfitted yourself for your adventure into the art of tai chi. But before you turn the page to begin your warm-ups, there's one more thing we suggest you do: have patience—with tai chi and with yourself.

When you watch people doing tai chi, it might seem easy, but when you start you'll soon become aware of the challenges tai chi presents. That's where the patience comes in. Immediate satisfaction may not happen. Don't be disappointed if you don't feel the picture of health after only a few days. And above all, don't expect perfection. Nobody does tai chi perfectly, and therein lies the ongoing challenge of the art.

As a beginner, you might feel strange or even awkward when doing tai chi, particularly if you are from a Western background and are used to fast-paced sports and moving in a straight line. Tai chi is slow, and its movements are curved and soft. The concept of internal power—the qi—might also seem foreign. But rest assured that once you get used to all these differences, you won't feel awkward. Instead you'll be hooked on these gentle movements that contain immense power. We suggest you give yourself at least three months to get used to these new concepts. Again, be patient.

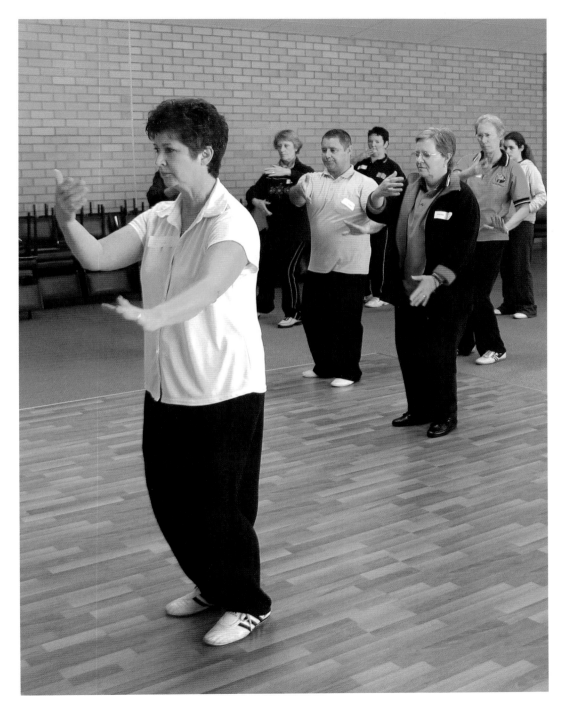

CHAPTER 3

THE SIX EASY STEPS

Over the years, Dr Lam and his colleagues have developed tai chi programs for beginners. The Six Easy Steps were created and tested by thousands of students and instructors who found them simple to follow and effective in improving health as well as building a solid foundation in tai chi.

Be sure to read Chapter 2 before starting this chapter. If you have any doubts regarding your physical condition, please consult your doctor before you start.

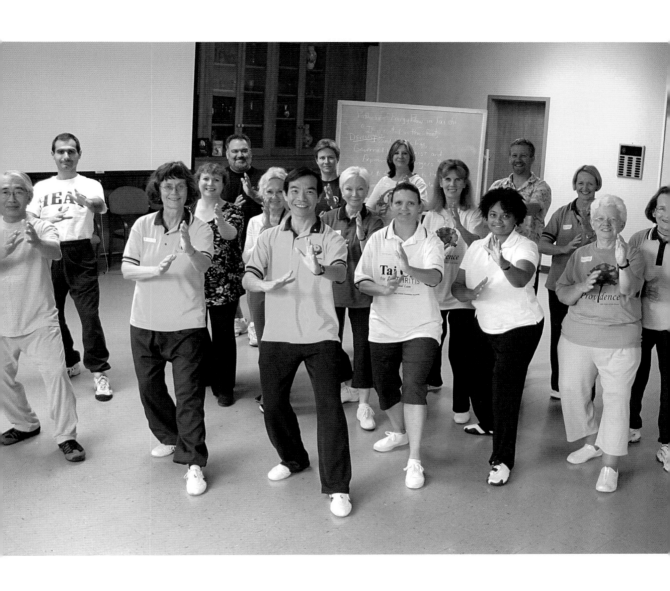

The Six Easy Steps are listed to the right. To help you remember them, we've designed Step 1 with *one* exercise; Step 2 with *two* stretches for each of the main parts of the body; Step 3 with *three* exercises, and so on. All the steps have the same number of exercises except for the last one.

Start by learning Steps 1–3, taking your time and practising until you're comfortable with these three steps. They're gentle, easy-to-remember stretching and cooling down exercises. When you are ready to advance beyond Step 3, keep in mind that you should always start with Steps 1 and 2 to warm up and prepare your body. You should finish with Step 3, cooling down.

From there on, throughout the rest of the steps, focus on the feel and rhythm of tai chi and don't worry too much about the details.

If you happen to have a physical disability that prevents you from doing the exercises and movements to the full range, follow the instructions only to the extent that allows you to remain within your comfort zone. If necessary, you can sit down and simply visualize yourself doing the movements to their full range. Let's say, for example, that you've suffered a stroke and can't move your left leg. Visualize that your left leg is moving to its full extent as you're sitting and moving other parts of your body. Studies have shown that people can improve their conditions with visualizations of this kind.

THE SIX EASY STEPS

Step 1
Warm-up One exercise to start the blood circulating.

Step 2
Stretching Two stretches for each of the main parts of the body.

Step 3
Cooling down Three exercises to do at the conclusion to enhance your flexibility and prevent injury.

Step 4
Qigong breathing Four exercises to cultivate inner energy.

Step 5
The Foundation Movements Five basic movements that will prepare you for your first sequences.

Step 6
The Tai Chi Beginner's Set A flowing sequence of movements that incorporates what you have learned so far.

In this chapter we have provided you with a lesson plan based on an hour-long lesson. If you have only half an hour or are unable to exercise for one hour because of your physical condition, do only part of the lesson.

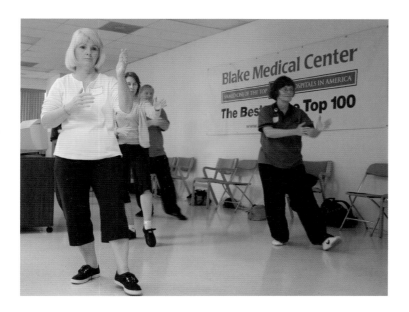

The plan is just a guide. Use your own discretion and adjust the plan according to your own physical ability and learning speed. Remember it's better to be slow and learn well rather than learn the entire program quickly and miss out on important principles. Also the length of time to exercise is not set in stone. Keep in mind that five minutes of exercise is better than none.

After learning new material, practise it for at least three sessions to become familiar, comfortable and proficient in the moves. Only then should you move on to the next lesson. Try to practise daily, or at least on most days of the week.

Lesson plan

After you've familiarized yourself with the first three steps, you can learn the steps in sequence. Or to make it more interesting, you can learn one qigong exercise from Step 4 and one movement from Step 5 during each lesson. If you find a movement difficult, do it in as many lessons as it feels right to you. Don't move on until you've practised and become familiar with what you've already studied.

It will take six to eight lessons (and at least three practice sessions for each lesson) to finish Steps 1 to 5. Having got to that stage, practise the first five steps for a while before moving on to the last step. It may then take another six to eight lessons to learn the last step.

You can continue to practise the Six Easy Steps for as long as you wish, in order to gain better health and reach a higher level of tai chi. After you've become proficient, probably after practising for a few months, you can move on to the 24 Forms in the second part of this book.

Step 1

Warm-up

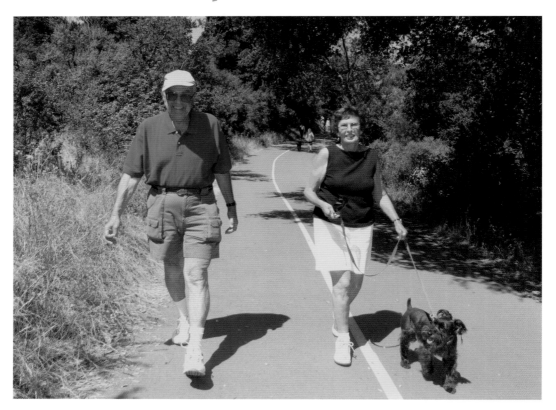

Choose one or more of the following:

* For approximately one or two minutes, walk around, gently shaking your hands and legs and clenching and unclenching your hands. This loosens your muscles and joints and starts the blood circulating in preparation for the exercises that follow.

* Give yourself a massage. First, rub your hands together. This makes them warm by increasing the qi. Then massage your legs, ankles and feet, and lower back and shoulders, rubbing your hands together intermittently.

* Take a short walk.

* Take a hot shower.

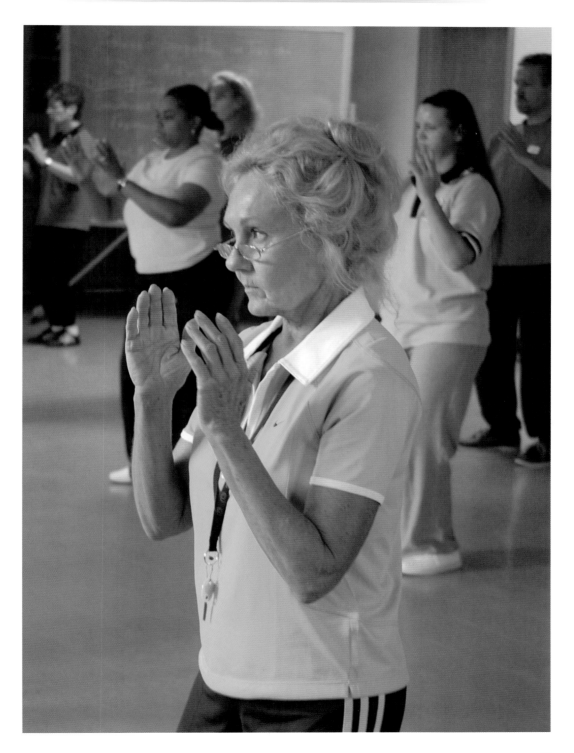

Step 2
Stretching

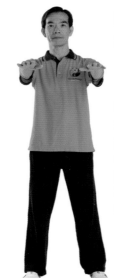

NECK
HEAD DOWN

Gently stretch six parts of the body—neck, shoulders, spine, hips, knees and ankles—with two stretches for each body part. It might help you to remember them by knowing we are working from the top down, starting with the neck, and ending at the ankles.

➊ As you inhale, bring both of your hands up slowly, imagining your wrists are being lifted by two balloons.

Practising these exercises regularly will enhance your flexibility and tone up your muscles. They were created with tai chi principles incorporated. At this stage, practise the outside shape as described below, and later in the book we will show you how to incorporate the tai chi principles. Keep the following guidelines in mind:

* Do all movements slowly, continuously and smoothly.
* Work within your comfort range. The first time you do a movement, stretch to only 70 per cent of your normal range then increase the range gradually after that.
* When appropriate, do both sides of the body.
* Do each stretch between three and five times. It doesn't matter which side you do first.

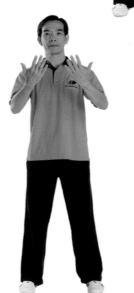

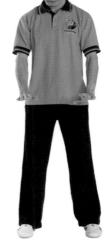

➋ Turn your palms to face you with your fingers pointing up. Bring them towards your chest, and push your chin (or your head) backwards gently.

➌ Exhaling, push both palms outwards, extending them in front of you, and then press your hands down slowly and gently. At the same time, slowly bring your head down towards your chest.

TURNING HEAD

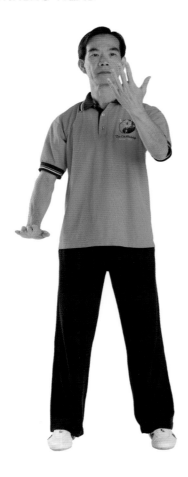

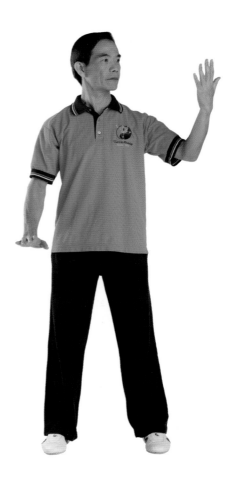

① Starting the same way as the previous exercise, lift up both hands. Then turn your left hand so that fingers are pointing up with the palm facing you. At the same time, gently push the right hand down so that it moves near the hip, with the palm facing down. Look at your left palm.

② Move your left hand to the left, turning your head slowly to the left and keeping your eyes on your palm. Now come back to face the front. Change palms so that your right palm is now facing you and the left is down near the left hip. Turn to the right while looking at the right palm.

Stretching

SHOULDERS
SHOULDER ROLL

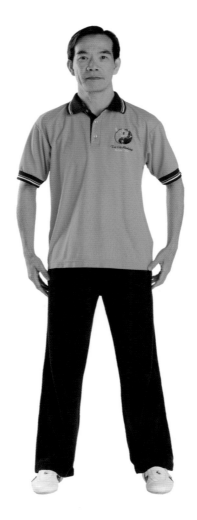

Roll your shoulders gently forward three times and then gently backwards three times.

GATHERING QI

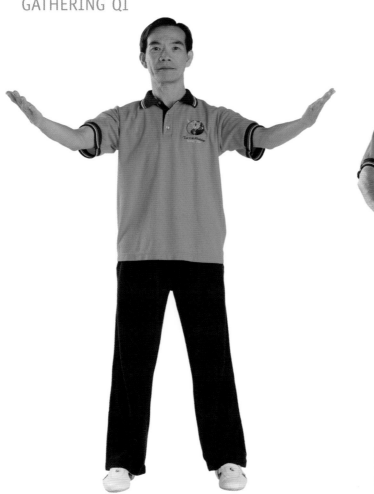

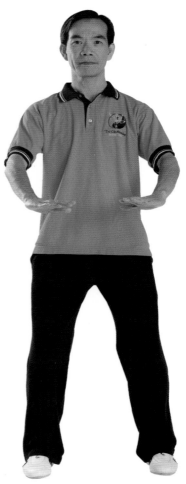

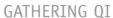

❶ Inhaling, extend your arms to the side, with the palms facing up, and move your arms upwards in a curve to above your head.

❷ As you exhale, gently press your hands down in front of your body to below your navel.

Stretching

SPINE
HEAVEN AND EARTH

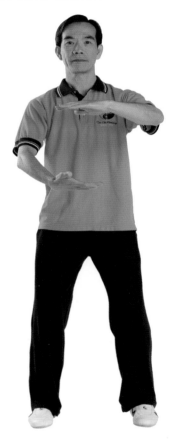

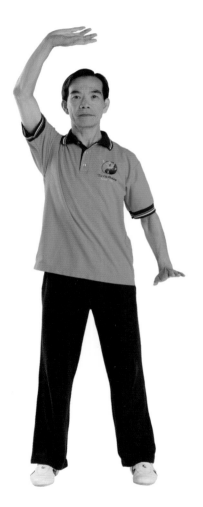

① Hold your hands in front of you, one above the other, as if you are carrying a large beach ball. Inhale.

② Exhaling, push one hand up as though your palm is pushing against the ceiling. At the same time, push the other hand down by your side, imagine stretching your spine gently. Then change hands and repeat the exercise.

SPINE TURN

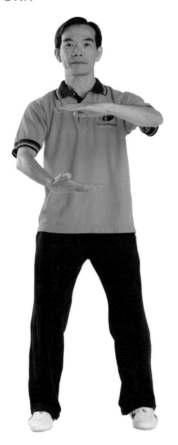 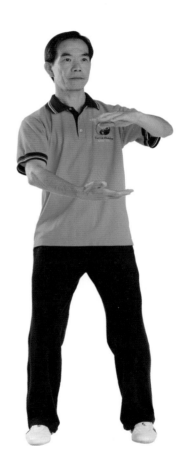

❶ Hold your hands in front of you, one above the other, as if you are carrying a large beach ball. Have the left hand on top.

❷ With your knees slightly bent, turn your waist gently to the left. Then change hands, putting the right hand on top and turn to the right. Keep your back upright and supple, and be sure to turn no more than 45 degrees from the front. Be sure also to turn your waist rather than twisting your shoulder to the sides.

Stretching

HIPS
FORWARD STRETCH

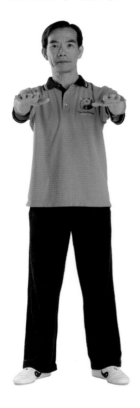 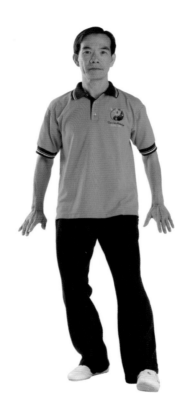 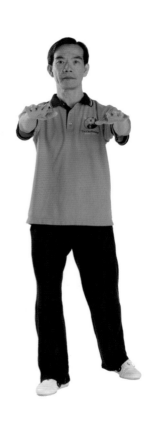

❶ Stand upright, and bring your hands up to shoulder height.

❷ Bend your knees slightly, and place your left heel out in front of you; push both hands back to help you balance.

❸ Step backwards so that your left foot is resting on the toes, while stretching your hands forward to about shoulder height for better balance. Repeat on the other side.

An easier alternative: Place your left foot parallel to the right foot before stepping backwards.

SIDE STRETCH

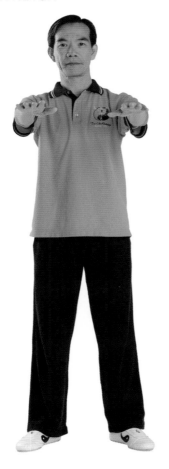

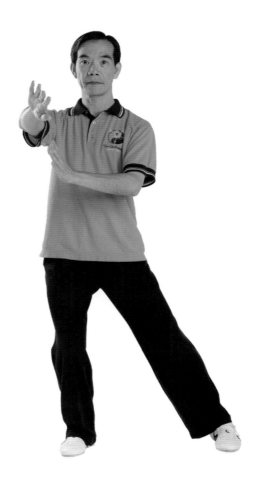

① Stand upright, and bring your hands up to shoulder height.

② Bending your knees slightly, push your hands to the side as though you're pushing against a wall. At the same time, stretch the opposite foot out sideways. Maintain an upright posture and stretch only as far as is comfortable.

Stretching

KNEES
KICK

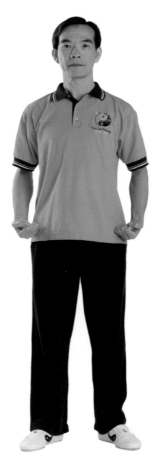

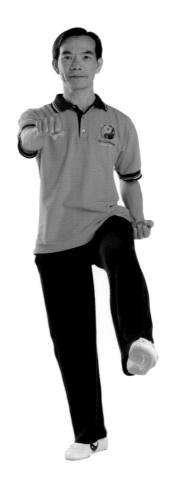

❶ Make loose fists, with the palm side up, and rest them at the sides of the hips. Bend your knees slightly.

❷ Stretch out one foot (like a kicking motion, but slowly and gently). At the same time, punch out gently with the opposite fist, turning it palm down. Bring your arm and leg back in and repeat on the other side.

STEP FORWARD

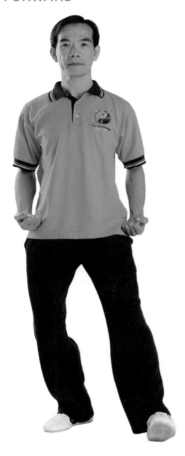

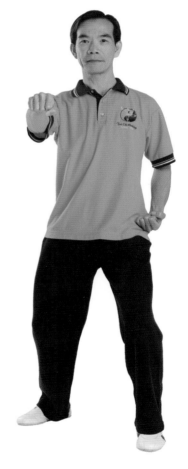

1 With your fists next to your hips as in the previous exercise, bend your knees slightly and step forward with one foot.

2 Shift your weight onto the front leg, and as your body moves forward, punch out with the opposite fist. Bring your foot back and do the same on the other side.

Stretching

ANKLES
TAPPING

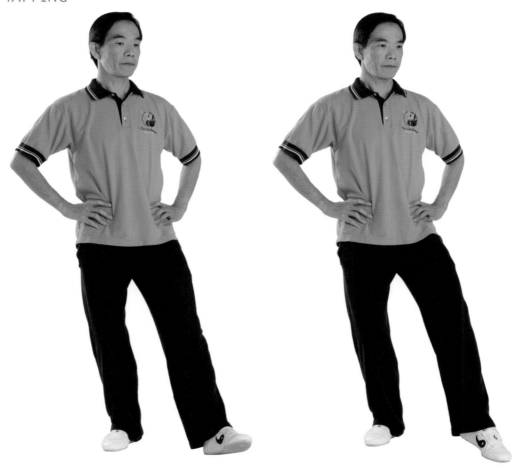

❶ Gently tap the floor with your heel.

❷ Gently tap the floor with your toes. Repeat heel and toes tap three times and then repeat with the other foot.

ROTATION

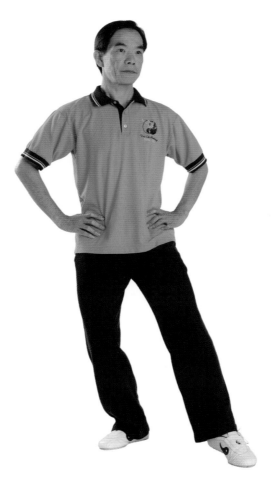

Lift up the heel of one foot, point the toes down and gently rotate your foot in one direction three times, and then in the other direction three times.
Repeat using the other foot.

An easier alternative:
Turn your foot inwards and outwards three times, avoiding over-stretching by not putting any weight on the turning foot. Repeat using the other foot.

Step 3
Cooling down

While these exercises are to be used after you complete your tai chi session, you should learn them now so that you can do them after your very first lesson. They will help to enhance your flexibility, relax your muscles and prevent injury.

PUNCHING THIGH

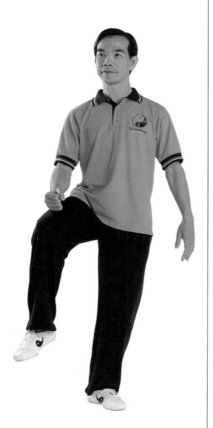

Lift your thigh to a comfortable height and gently punch it. Repeat with the other leg.

TENSE AND RELAX

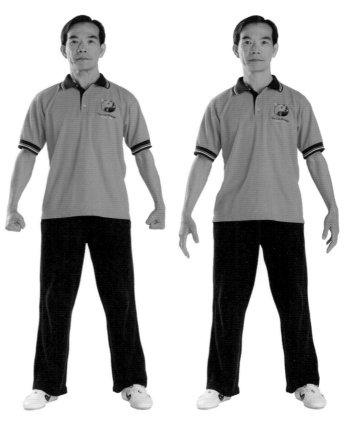

❶ Inhaling, clench your hands, gently contract the muscles of your body, and stand on your toes if you can.

❷ Exhale, letting everything relax.

GATHERING QI

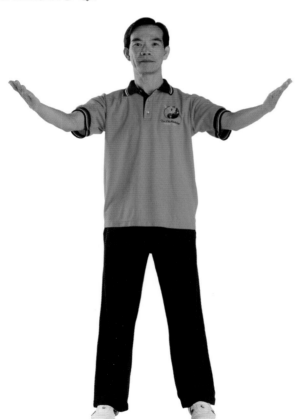

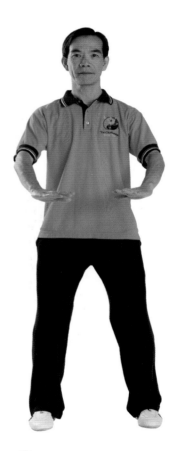

① Inhaling, extend your arms to the side, with the palms facing up, and move your arms upwards in a curve above your head.

② As you exhale, gently press your palms down in front of your body to just below your navel.

Step 4
Qigong breathing

One of the oldest exercises in Chinese history, dating back more than 2000 years, qigong (pronounced "chee-gung") encompasses a variety of breathing, gymnastic and meditative exercises. The word "qigong" is a combination of the words "qi" and "gong". In Chinese, *qi* means several things, the most common being "air". But in the field of Chinese medicine and tai chi, *qi* means "the life energy inside a person". This life energy comes from the combination of three components: the air we breathe into our lungs; the qi that we already have when we are born; and the qi we absorb from food and water through the digestive system. Qi circulates throughout the body, performing many functions that contribute to the maintenance of good health.

Gong means "a method of exercise that requires a great deal of time to do well". Qigong is thus a method of cultivating qi, but one that takes a long time in order to become proficient.

We integrate these ancient concepts of nature into the following four qigong exercises. The exercises are easy to learn and at first may appear too simple. Don't be fooled by this initial appearance. Continue to practise them regularly and you'll realize their depth and application. They enhance breath control, relaxation and healing, and are designed to cultivate your vital inner energy, which will enhance your level of tai chi.

Note: Do the following exercises slowly, holding the postures as long as you feel comfortable. As you progress, you'll be able to sustain the positions longer. When practising them, keep your mouth closed, but not tightly, with your tongue lightly touching the upper palate. Breathe in and out through your nose (unless you have difficulty breathing through your nose).

THE POSTURE OF INFINITY

In Chinese, this posture is called *wu ji*, which means "infinite" or "never ending". Ancient Chinese philosophers believed that the universe originated in a state of *wu ji*, and the Posture of Infinity emulates this state. It encourages posture awareness, which is a fundamental part of tai chi and vital to your getting a good start. The upright posture helps the body function in the most effective way, minimizing the wearing of joints, ligaments and muscles, and protecting the internal organs. Most important, it enhances the flow of qi and internal power, thus strengthening the internal structures.

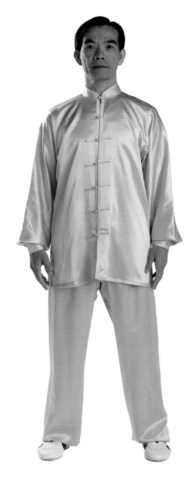

VALID PROOF

At the beginning of a qigong or tai chi session, spend one minute in the Posture of Infinity, checking your body for tension and weakness. Then cleanse your mind. At the end of the session, repeat this and check your body and mind to see if you're more relaxed and in better control of your body and mind. If you are, you'll realize how your body and mind have changed for the better.

Stand upright but relaxed, with your feet shoulder-width apart. Look straight ahead, tuck in your chin, and make sure your shoulders, elbows and knees are relaxed. Imagine your body as a string that is being stretched gently from both ends. Cleanse your mind. Focus on the correct posture: upright without tension.

Qigong breathing

THE POSTURE OF TAI CHI

From *wu ji*, the universe developed into a state of *tai ji*, or tai chi, which means "vastness" or "infinity". This exercise focuses on being aware of your dan tian, an area approximately three fingerwidths below your navel. It's called the "storage house of the qi", and it's the centre of gravity and life energy. Awareness of this area will enhance the cultivation of qi, help you to maintain the right posture, and strengthen inner structures, such as the deep stabilizing muscles. Also called the core muscles, the deep stabilizing muscles are the muscles closest to the spine. Recent studies have shown that they support and strengthen the spine, and play a vital role in back stability.

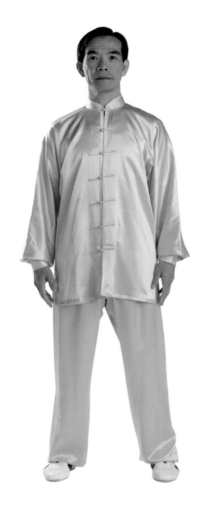

❶ Start with the Posture of Infinity (see page 51).

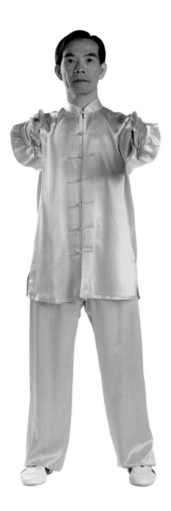

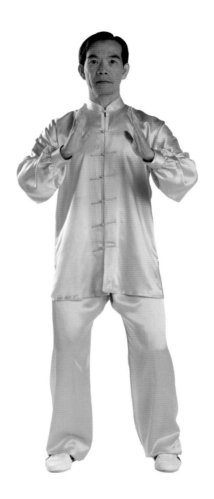

2 As you inhale, slowly bring your hands up to chest height, with the palms facing each other.

3 Bring your hands towards your chest, bending your knees slightly, and exhale. In this position, focus on your dan tian. When you feel a little tired, stretch your hands out as in the previous posture. Bring your hands down and slowly stand up.

Qigong breathing

THE POSTURE OF OPENING AND CLOSING

This posture symbolizes the separation of tai chi into yin and yang. Tai chi is the combination of yin and yang, which are complete polar opposites yet complementary to each other. When both yin and yang are well balanced and in harmony, qi is abundant and strong. Breathing awareness is the purpose of this exercise. Breathing is central to all qigong exercises and a fundamental part of tai chi. This is one of the most powerful exercises to enhance qi. It's the cornerstone of Sun-style tai chi, recognized for its effective cultivation of qi.

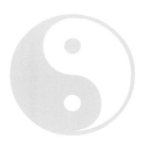

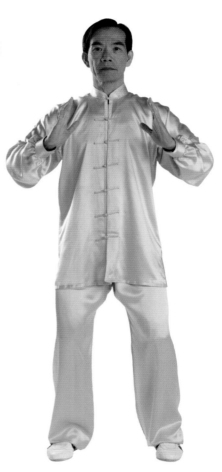

❶ Continuing from the end of the previous posture, inhale and slowly pull your hands apart to shoulder width. If your knees feel tired, gently straighten them.

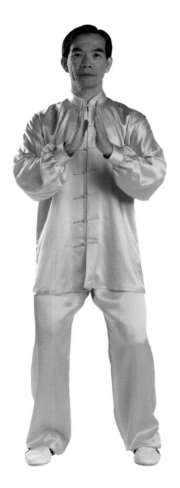

This exercise demonstrates the working of yin and yang. Closing is yin and opening is yang. To start with, do this exercise no more than three times, then more frequently as you become stronger. (While it's customary to do these exercises in increments of three, it's all right for our purposes to make the increments smaller.) As you breathe in and out, imagine there is a gentle magnetic force between your palms. Pull against this resistance as you breathe in and push against it as you breathe out.

ABDOMINAL BREATHING METHOD

This breathing method enhances qi and promotes relaxation. Imagine that, as you breathe, the air travels through your nose and down your trachea (airway to the lungs), filling the lungs and then the abdomen. As your abdomen fills with air, it bulges gently outwards. As you breathe out, the abdomen contracts. Picture in your mind the air expelling from the abdomen, lungs, trachea and, finally, through your nose. (In reality, air doesn't enter the abdomen; this is simply a visualization technique to help you utilize your diaphragm to open up more air space in your lungs.) Practise this breathing method as often as you can. You can do it almost anywhere.

❷ Exhaling, gently push your hands towards each other, bringing them as close to each other as possible without touching. If you've straightened your knees, gently bend them again. Continue opening and closing your hands several times. Complete the exercise by stretching your hands forward and returning to the Posture of Infinity, straightening your knees.

Qigong breathing

THE POSTURE OF YIN-YANG HARMONY

This exercise is designed to mobilize and cultivate qi. As qi circulates through the body, it grows stronger, and as your tai chi level improves, you'll be able to direct and mobilize qi more effectively. This will enhance your flow and effectively improve inner power. Keep your palms facing each other throughout this exercise.

When you breathe in, visualize your qi moving up to the middle of your chest. When you breathe out, visualize your qi moving down to the dan tian. It doesn't matter if you don't feel or know what qi is. Simply think about the dan tian as you breathe in and out. As your tai chi improves, you'll be able to feel the qi. While the sensation of qi varies from person to person, for most people it feels like a warm and slightly heavy sensation. Whether or not you can feel the qi, you will improve your internal energy through practice.

Note: You don't have to feel any qi before moving on to the next step. As long as you're familiar with these postures and breathing patterns, you can move on.

MAKING QIGONG WORK FOR YOU

Practise these qigong exercises as often as you can. You can also use a variation when sitting (for example, when sitting down waiting for a doctor's appointment): sit straight, cleanse your mind, use abdominal breathing and centre yourself. When you're anxious or getting angry, try to focus on your breathing and posture and feel your qi. It will help you relax and get more enjoyment out of life.

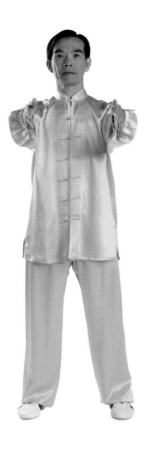

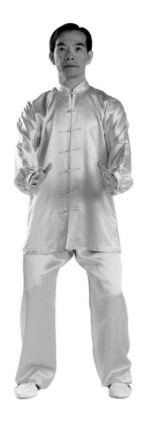

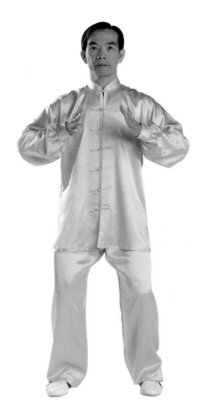

① As you inhale, slowly bring your hands up to chest height.

② Exhaling, bring your hands down, then towards your body.

③ Again inhaling, bring your hands up to your chest. Continue moving your arms in a loop as the diagram below shows. Stand up as you breathe in and bend your knees as you breathe out.

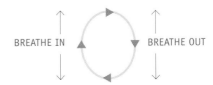

BREATHE IN   BREATHE OUT

Step 5
The Foundation Movements

These five movements are designed to provide you with a good foundation for tai chi. They will make your next step easier and more enjoyable. At this point, don't think about the martial application of tai chi; instead, focus on developing a soft, yet powerful, internal force. To do this, concentrate on using the minimum strength necessary to execute all the movements, and follow our instructions as closely as possible within your physical ability.

Instead of limiting yourself to doing the left and right side only once, you can continue to do both sides for as many times as you're comfortable. We recommend practising each movement three to five times before bringing both feet together to finish off.

Once you are familiar with each movement, try to incorporate the mental state you've reached from the qigong exercises of Step 4. This will help improve your concentration, internal tai chi component and your level of tai chi.

Movement 1
STEPPING FORWARD

This movement will help you transfer your weight from one leg to another in the appropriate tai chi way—an important component of tai chi essential principles.

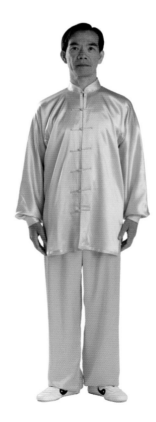

❶ Stand upright with your toes pointing out. Imagine your torso is a string, being gently stretched from both ends. Keep your shoulders down, and release any tension in your body.

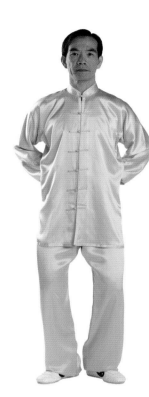

2 Bend your knees slightly while maintaining an upright body.

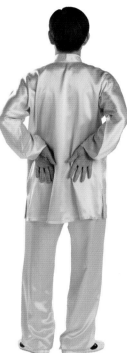

3 Bring your hands to the back, palms facing out. Note that your hands rest on the small of your back, where there are acupuncture (energy) points, to enhance your qi.

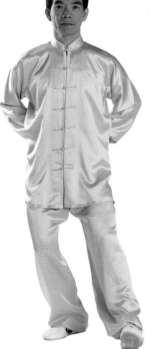

4 Shift your weight onto the right foot. Take a step forward with your left foot, placing the heel down first. Touch down like a cat.

The Foundation Movements

STEPPING FORWARD

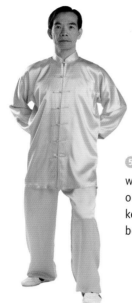

5 Now shift your weight forward onto the left foot, keeping your body upright.

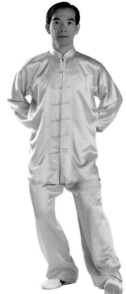

6 Shift your weight back onto the right foot, allowing the toes of the left foot to point upwards.

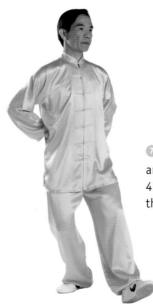

7 Turn your body and your toes 45 degrees to the left.

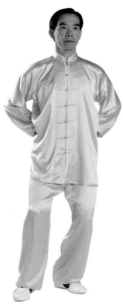

8 Shift your weight onto the left foot, placing the ball of your right foot near the left, with a comfortable distance between them to maintain good balance.

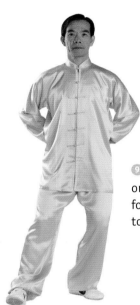

9 Step forward onto your right foot, with the toes pointing up.

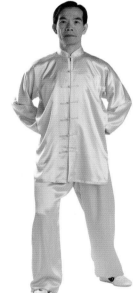

10 Shift your weight forward onto your right foot.

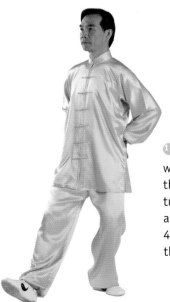

11 Shift your weight back onto the left foot, then turn your body and right foot 45 degrees to the right.

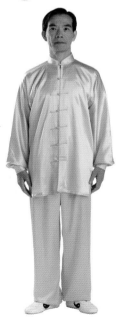

12 Bring your left foot near the right and then stand back up in the starting position.

The Foundation Movements

Movement 2
PARTING THE WILD HORSE'S MANE

This movement integrates weight transference with posture and dan tian awareness.

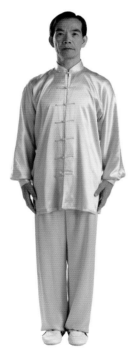 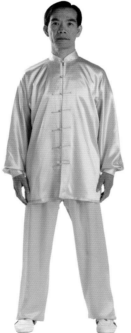 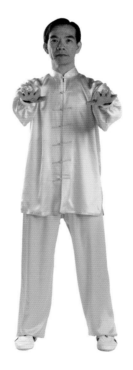 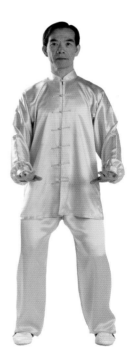

❶ Stand upright without tension.

❷ Lift up your left foot, and place it so that your feet are shoulder-width apart.

❸ Inhaling, slowly lift your arms and hands (palms facing down) to chest height. Imagine both wrists are tied to a balloon that is gently lifting up your hands.

❹ Exhaling, press your hands down gently, bending your knees slightly.

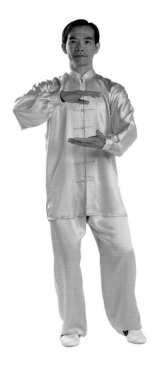

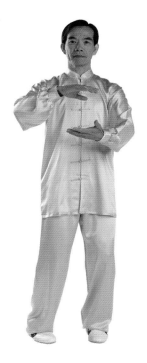

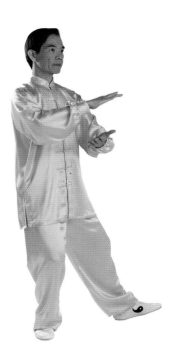

⑤ Bring your right hand up over your left palm as though you were carrying a large beach ball. Be sure there is a space between your hands and your body. Imagine there's an energy field between them. Put your weight on the right foot, placing the left foot (ball of the foot only) close to the right.

An easier alternative: If you find it difficult to keep your weight on the right leg while stepping to the left, turn your right toes inwards about 45 degrees before you move, as shown above. You can use this option for other, similar movements.

⑥ Keeping your weight on the right foot, step out to the left with your left foot, with the heel on the ground and the toes up. Bring your hands slightly closer to each other.

The Foundation Movements
PARTING THE WILD HORSE'S MANE

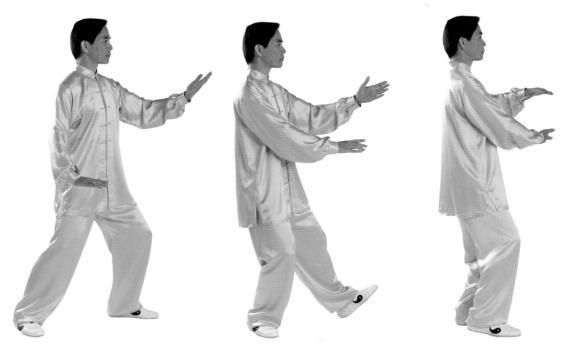

7 Shift your weight forward to form a bow stance, and separate your hands.

8 Shift your weight back to the right, bringing your hands slightly closer to you. Turn body and foot 45 degrees to the left.

9 Put the weight back on your left foot, bring your right foot near the left. Place your hands as if carrying a ball, left hand on top.

THE BOW STANCE

A stance is the position of your lower body. A bow stance, as in position 7 on this page, is a position in which one can deliver force from a stable and strong position. The foot at the front is pointing straight ahead, with 70 per cent of the weight resting on it. Imagine there's a line between the kneecap and outer border of the toes. To avoid over-bending the knee, the knee should not go past this vertical line. As a beginner, you'll find it easier to at first bend just a little and then gradually increase the degree of your bend. The back leg should be bent very slightly, with 30 per cent of your weight resting on the foot and the toes pointing out at 45 degrees. The feet should be shoulder-width apart.

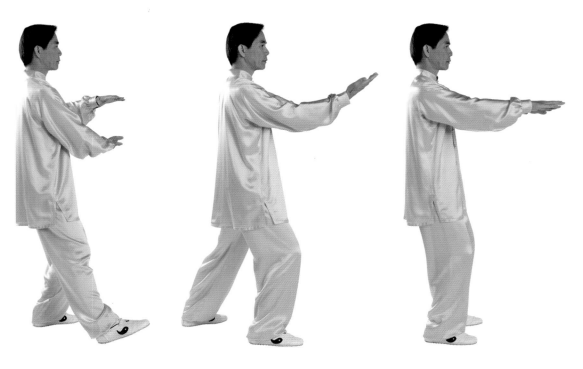

⑩ Step forward with the right foot, heel first.

⑪ Shift your weight forward to the right, separating your hands.

⑫ Bring your left foot near the right foot, and hold both hands stretched out in front of you. Bring your hands down and slowly stand up.

The Foundation Movements

Movement 3
BRUSH KNEE

This movement is similar to the previous one, and will reinforce your knowledge of it.

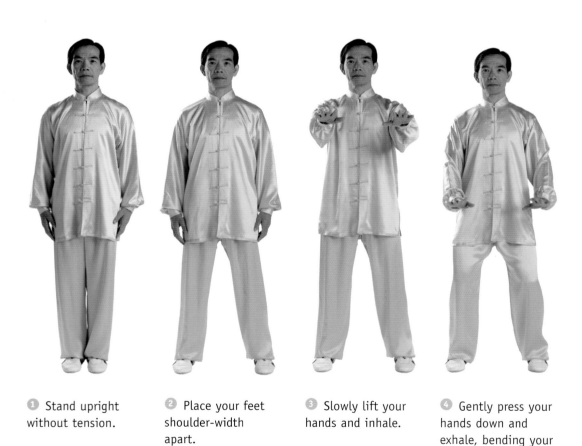

❶ Stand upright without tension.

❷ Place your feet shoulder-width apart.

❸ Slowly lift your hands and inhale.

❹ Gently press your hands down and exhale, bending your knees slightly.

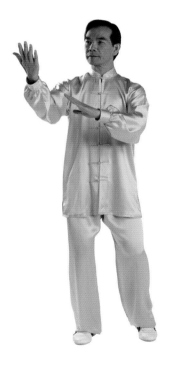 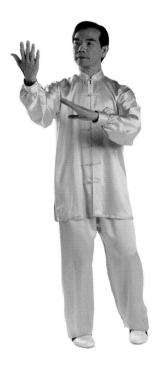

⑤ Stretch your right hand out, and place your left hand next to the right elbow. Have your weight on the right, bringing the left foot closer to the right.

An easier alternative: If you find it difficult to step out to the left, for the next step turn the right toe inwards about 45 degrees, as shown above.

The Foundation Movements

BRUSH KNEE

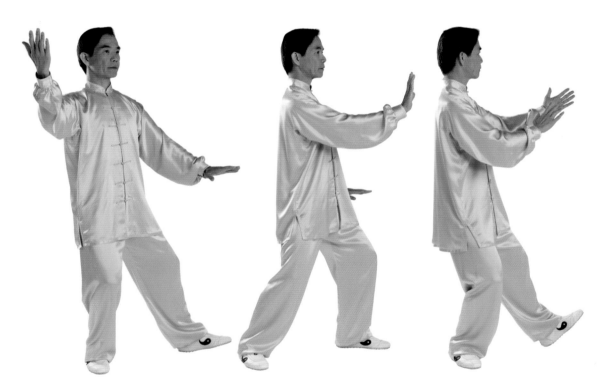

6 Step out to the left with the left foot, stretching your right hand slightly upwards, and bringing your left hand downwards.

7 Shift your weight forward onto the left foot. Move the left hand past the knee to be near the left hip as you slowly push the right hand forward.

8 Shift your weight backwards, bringing your hands back. Turn your body and left foot 45 degrees to the left.

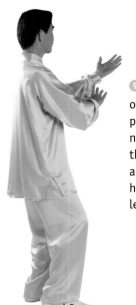

⑨ Put your weight onto the left foot, placing the right foot near the left. Stretch the left hand out, and place the right hand next to the left elbow.

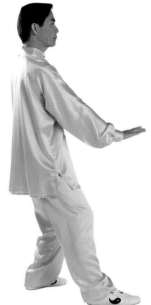

⑩ Step forward with your right foot. Separate your hands.

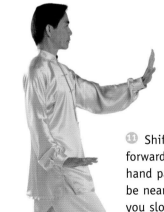

⑪ Shift your weight forward. Bring the right hand past the knee to be near the right hip as you slowly push the left hand forward.

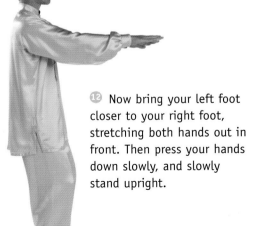

⑫ Now bring your left foot closer to your right foot, stretching both hands out in front. Then press your hands down slowly, and slowly stand upright.

The Foundation Movements

Movement 4
STEPPING BACKWARDS

This movement will prepare you for the next movement, Repulse the Monkey, a more difficult sequence.

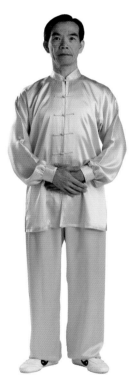 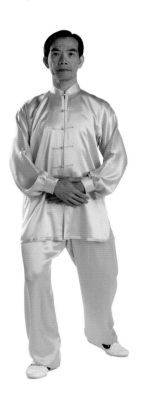 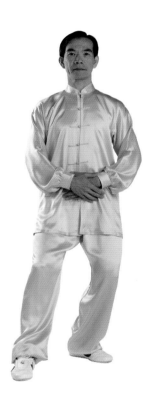

❶ Stand upright with your hands over your lower abdomen, just below the navel. (According to ancient Chinese tradition, to take advantage of the complementary yin and yang, men should place their left hand on the abdomen first, and women should place their right first.)

❷ Bend your knees slightly. Putting your weight on the right foot, step back with the left, placing the foot at a 45 degree angle and touching the floor lightly with the ball of the foot first.

❸ Shift your weight back onto the left foot, keeping your body upright. Lift your right heel and adjust your foot so that your toes are facing forward.

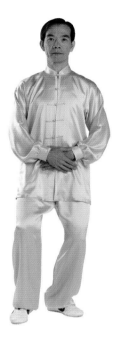

④ Moving inwards in a gentle curve, bring your right foot closer to your left foot without putting any weight on it.

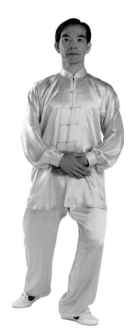

⑤ Move the right foot backwards and outwards in a gentle curve.

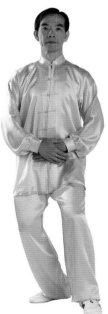

⑥ Shift your weight back onto your right foot.

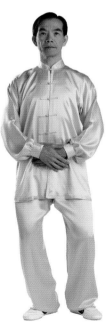

⑦ Lift up your left heel and straighten the toes of that foot to face forward, and then bring your left foot back to join your right. Then slowly stand up.

The Foundation Movements

Movement 5
REPULSE THE MONKEY—UPPER BODY ONLY

To make this complex movement easier to grasp, we are going to learn the movements of the upper part of the body first. Practise for a while until you are familiar with it, then combine the upper body movements with Movement 4, Stepping Backwards, for the entire sequence.

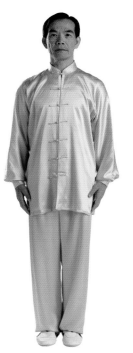 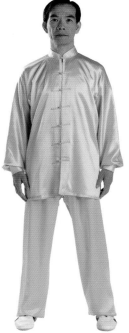 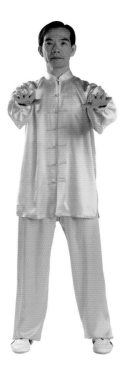 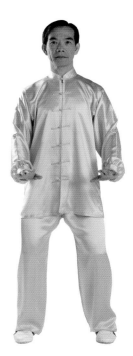

❶ Stand upright without any tension in the body.

❷ Move your left foot so that your feet are shoulder-width apart.

❸ Slowly lift your hands.

❹ Press your hands down gently, bending your knees slightly.

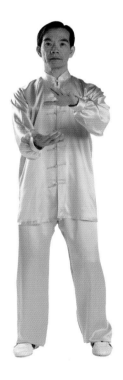

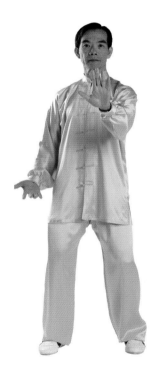

⑤ Bring both hands in front of your chest as though you're carrying a small ball, with the left hand on top and the fingers pointing forward.

⑥ Gently push your left hand forward, with the palm facing outwards, and bring the right hand back near the hip, with the palm facing upwards.

The Foundation Movements
REPULSE THE MONKEY—UPPER BODY ONLY

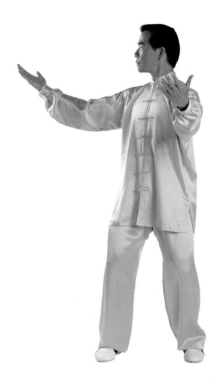 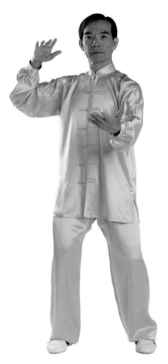 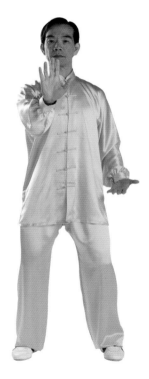

⑦ Turning your body to the right, bring your right hand up, turning the palm slightly. Look at your right hand. Both palms are now facing each other diagonally, as though they were communicating with each other.

⑧ Start to turn your head back to the front while you bring your right hand next to your ear and your left hand back slightly.

⑨ Push your right hand forward while bringing your left hand, palm upwards, back near your left hip.

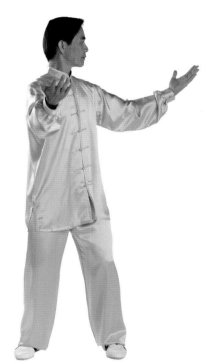

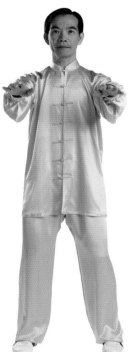

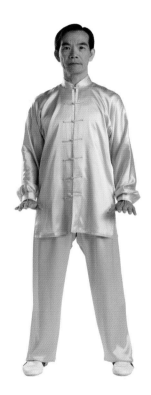

⑩ Turn your body to the left, turning your right palm upwards and bringing your left hand back.

⑪ Push your left hand forward, turn the right palm downward and stretch both hands forward.

⑫ Slowly press both your hands down and stand up.

The Foundation Movements

REPULSE THE MONKEY—THE COMPLETE MOVEMENT

Now you will combine the upper body movements with Movement 4, Stepping Backwards. First follow the upper body movement steps 1–7, then do the following.

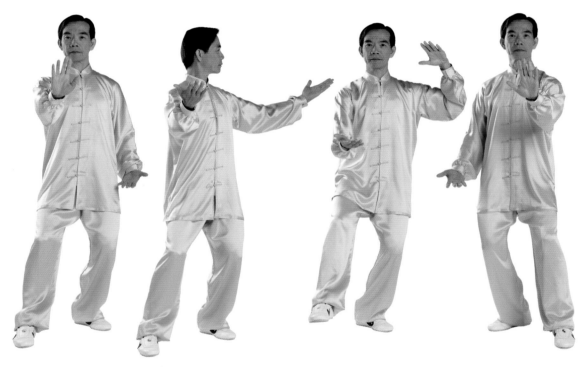

❶ As you push your right hand forward, step back with your left foot and shift your weight onto your left.

❷ Turn your body to the left, left hand up. Turn both palms up.

❸ Bringing your left hand near your ear and your right hand back slightly, begin to lift up your right foot.

❹ Step back with your right foot, pushing your left hand forward and pulling the right hand back, while putting all your weight on the right foot. Adjust your left toes so that the foot is pointing forward.

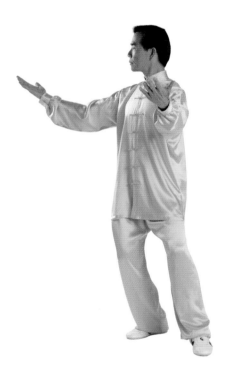

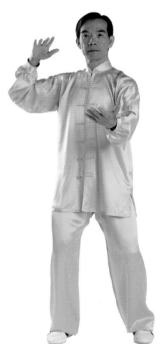

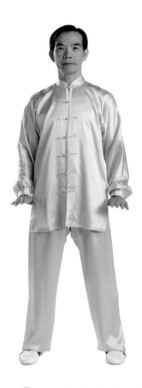

5 Turn your body to the right, right hand up. Turn left palm up.

6 Bringing your right hand near your ear and your left hand back, palm turning in, bring your left foot back near your right foot.

7 Stretch both hands forward in front of the chest, shoulder-width apart, and then slowly press both your hands down and stand up.

Congratulations! You've done the five steps. Practise until you're completely comfortable with them before you move on to Step 6, where you'll join all the movements into a tai chi set.

Step 6

The Tai Chi Beginner's Set

This step is a combination of all the movements and qigong exercises that you've learned so far, plus several new movements. Learn one move, or at the most two, at a time. Practise each until you're comfortable with it before moving on to the next one. During the learning phase, finish off each session with a closing movement, as you have done previously, by bringing your hands slowly down as you stand up.

Sometimes, trying too hard to cultivate qi can make you tense and produce a counterproductive effect. At this point, simply understanding the concept of qi is enough. You'll feel it gradually, and it may take a while, so don't worry. The key to cultivating qi and improving in tai chi is to follow the essential principles, which we'll provide as we go (there's also a summary of these principles in Chapter 4). Whether or not you feel the qi, your qi will grow stronger, your health will benefit and with practice, you'll progress towards better tai chi.

Don't worry too much about the timing of your breathing—when to inhale, when to exhale—for a while either. That, too, will come in time. Breathe naturally, and within your comfort zone, and follow our breathing instructions wherever provided. Don't force anything. Keep practising and the right feel will come to you in time.

It may take between six and eight lessons to learn the entire set of movements. When you've completed them all, we suggest regular practice of the four qigong exercises (Step 4) followed by the complete Tai Chi Beginner's Set for a few weeks (be sure to warm up and cool down at each practice session) before starting the next part, the 24 Forms. How many different sets of forms you learn isn't important. What *is* important is to study and stick to the essential principles of tai chi (see p. 112). That way, you'll soon progress and gain the consequent enjoyment and health benefits.

The movements of the Tai Chi Beginner's Set are as follows (please note the numbering of this set is different from Step 5):

1 Commencement
2 Parting the Wild Horse's Mane (left, right, left)
3 White Crane Flashing Wings
4 Brush Knee (left, right, left)
5 Playing the Lute
6 Repulse the Monkey (left, right, left, right)
7 Closing

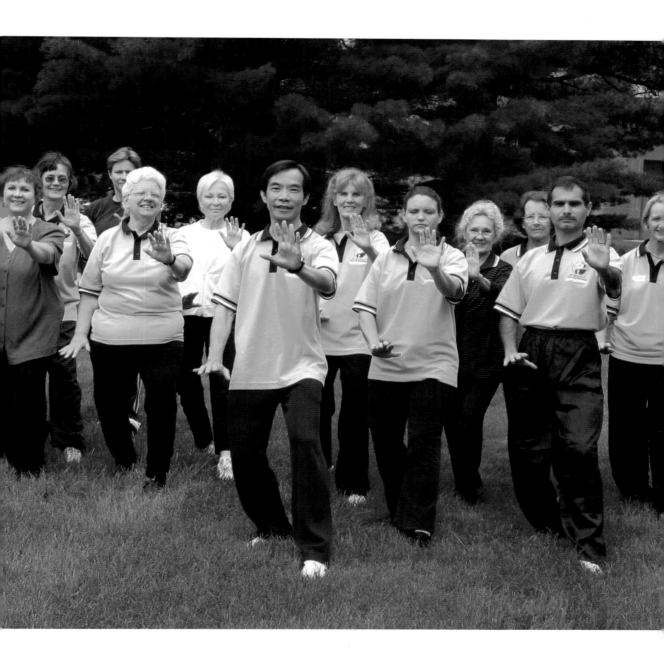

✶ =TAI CHI FOR BETTER BALANCE,

The Tai Chi Beginner's Set

Movement 1
COMMENCEMENT

From now on, whenever a position or direction might be ambiguous, we'll give you a clock position for precision. For instance, straight ahead is 12 o'clock, moving to the right is 3 o'clock, moving backwards or behind you is 6 o'clock, and moving to the left is 9 o'clock. Midway between directly ahead and to your right—in other words, at a 45-degree angle—is 1.30; 45 degrees to the left is 10.30.

We start facing 12 o'clock.

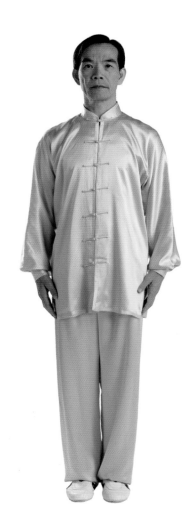

❶ Stand upright without tension.

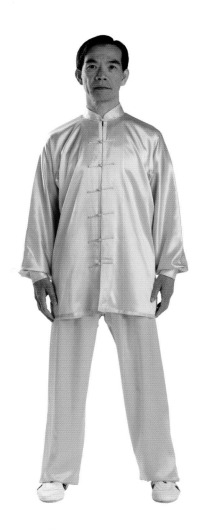 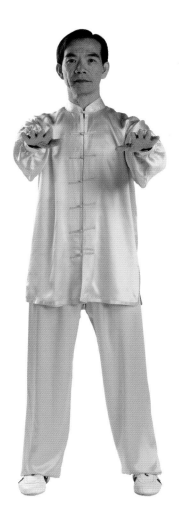 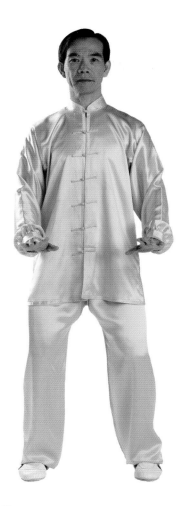

② Lift up your left foot, and place it so your feet are shoulder-width apart.

③ Inhaling, slowly lift your arms and hands, with the palms facing down, to chest height.

④ Exhaling, press your hands down gently, bending your knees slightly.

The Tai Chi Beginner's Set

Movement 2
PARTING THE WILD HORSE'S MANE

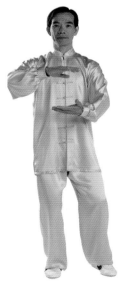

1 Bring your right hand up over your left palm as though carrying a large beach ball. Put your weight on the right foot, placing the left foot (ball of the foot only) close to the right.

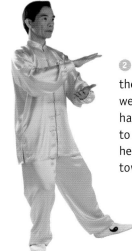

2 Move your left heel to the left without putting weight on it. Bring your hands slightly closer to each other. Your left heel should be pointing towards 9 o'clock.

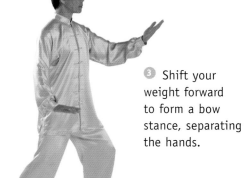

3 Shift your weight forward to form a bow stance, separating the hands.

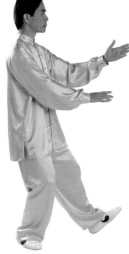

4 Shift your weight back to the right, bringing your hands slightly closer to you. Turn body and left foot 45 degrees to the left.

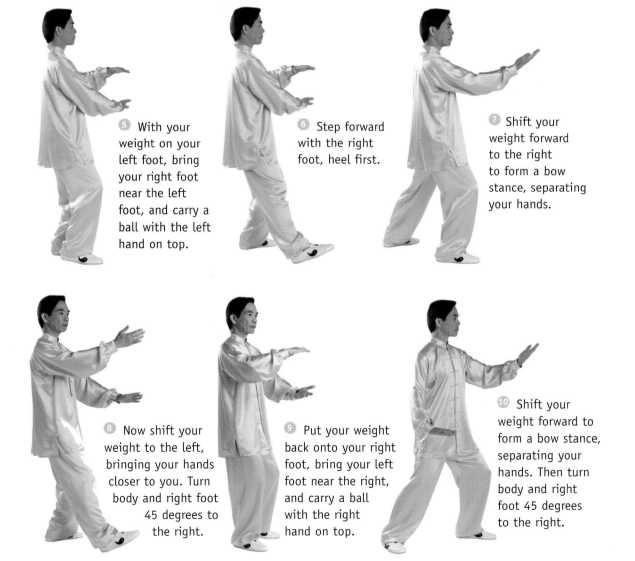

5 With your weight on your left foot, bring your right foot near the left foot, and carry a ball with the left hand on top.

6 Step forward with the right foot, heel first.

7 Shift your weight forward to the right to form a bow stance, separating your hands.

8 Now shift your weight to the left, bringing your hands closer to you. Turn body and right foot 45 degrees to the right.

9 Put your weight back onto your right foot, bring your left foot near the right, and carry a ball with the right hand on top.

10 Shift your weight forward to form a bow stance, separating your hands. Then turn body and right foot 45 degrees to the right.

The Tai Chi Beginner's Set

Movement 3
✕ WHITE CRANE FLASHING WINGS

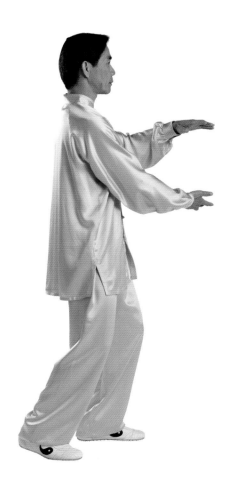

❶ With your weight on your left foot, step forward with your right foot about half a step. Turn the left palm down and the right palm up. Move both hands closer, ending with the left hand over the right hand, palms opposite each other as if you were carrying a ball.

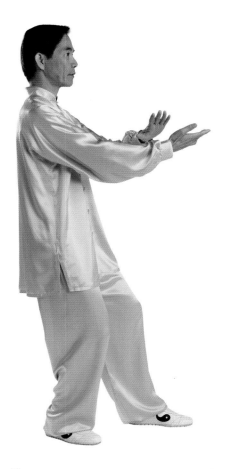

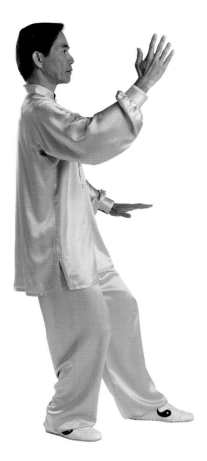

② Shift your weight back on the right foot. Bring your hands towards the right, moving them closer together, as if you were partially compressing the ball.

③ With your weight resting on your back (right) foot, bring your right hand up, palm in, left palm down, as shown, and bring your left foot back slightly, resting on the ball of the foot.

The Tai Chi Beginner's Set

Movement 4
BRUSH KNEE

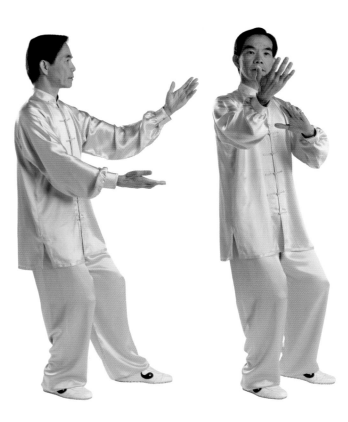

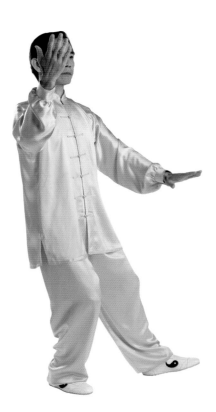

1 Turn your body to the left slightly and then to the right, moving your right hand down in a curve and then to the right, and your left hand up and then to the right.

2 Stretch your right hand out, and bring your left hand next to the right elbow. Have your weight on the right foot, bringing the left foot closer to the right.

3 Step towards the left with the left foot (towards 9 o'clock), stretching your right hand slightly upwards, and bringing your left hand downwards.

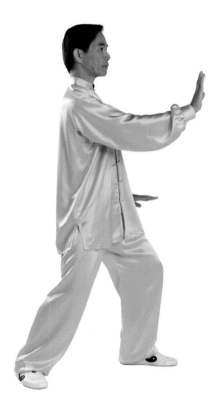 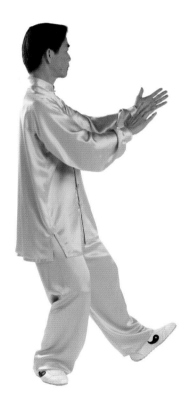

4 Shift your weight forward. The left hand moves back past the knee to be near the left hip as the right hand slowly pushes forward.

5 Shift your weight back onto the right foot, bringing your hands back. Turn your body and left foot 45 degrees to the left.

The Tai Chi Beginner's Set

BRUSH KNEE

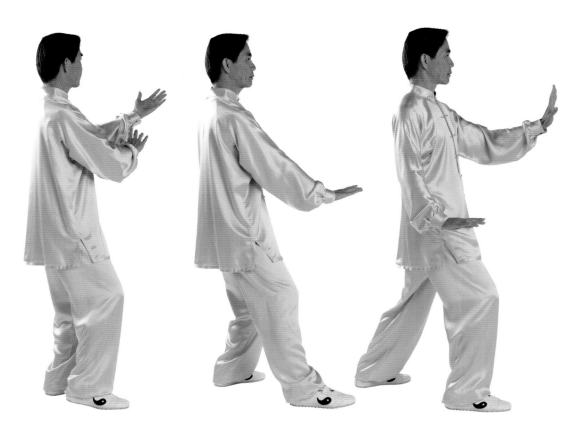

6 Put your weight onto the left foot, placing the right foot near the left. Stretch the left hand out to the left, and bring your right hand next to the left elbow.

7 Step to the right with your right foot (towards 9 o'clock), stretching your left hand slightly upwards and bringing your right hand downwards.

8 Shift your weight forward. The right hand moves back past the knee to be near the right hip as the left hand slowly pushes forward.

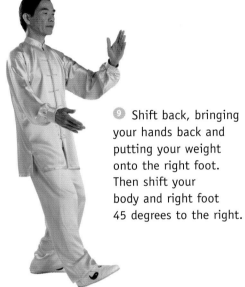

9 Shift back, bringing your hands back and putting your weight onto the right foot. Then shift your body and right foot 45 degrees to the right.

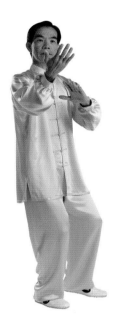

10 Stretch the right hand out, placing your left hand next to the right elbow. Have your weight on the right foot, bringing the left foot closer to the right.

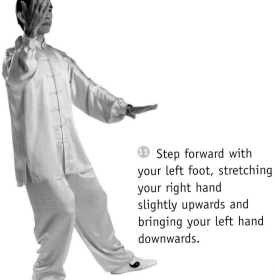

11 Step forward with your left foot, stretching your right hand slightly upwards and bringing your left hand downwards.

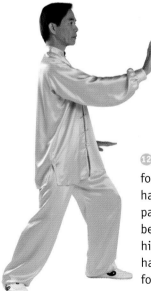

12 Shift your weight forward. The left hand moves back past the knee to be near the left hip as the right hand slowly pushes forward.

The Tai Chi Beginner's Set

Movement 5
PLAYING THE LUTE

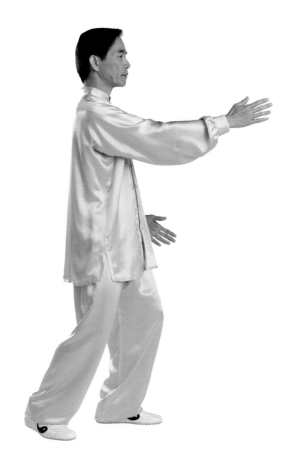

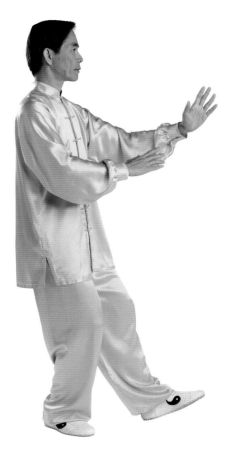

❶ Take a half step forward with your right foot, and push your right hand forward slightly.

❷ Shift your weight back onto the right foot. Slowly turn both palms to face inwards and at the same time bring your right hand back and push your left hand forward. At the same time, bring your left foot forward slightly to rest on the heel, without placing any weight on it.

Movement 6
REPULSE THE MONKEY

Do a sequence of four of these movements, as follows.

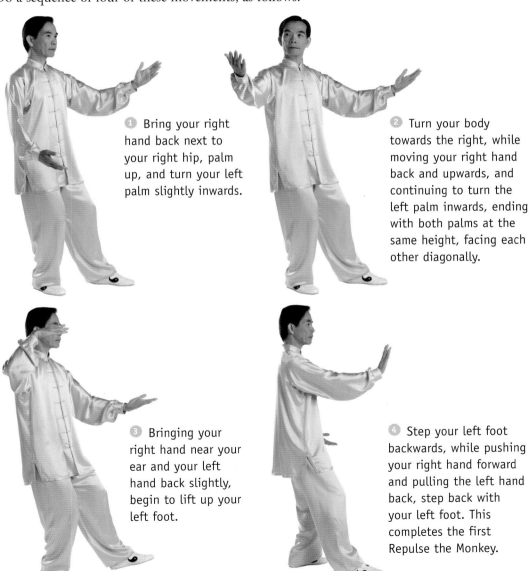

① Bring your right hand back next to your right hip, palm up, and turn your left palm slightly inwards.

② Turn your body towards the right, while moving your right hand back and upwards, and continuing to turn the left palm inwards, ending with both palms at the same height, facing each other diagonally.

③ Bringing your right hand near your ear and your left hand back slightly, begin to lift up your left foot.

④ Step your left foot backwards, while pushing your right hand forward and pulling the left hand back, step back with your left foot. This completes the first Repulse the Monkey.

The Tai Chi Beginner's Set
REPULSE THE MONKEY

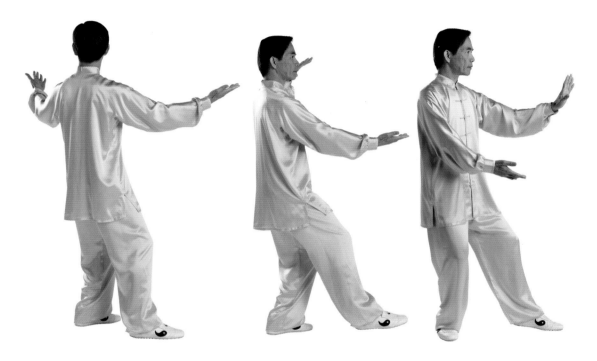

❺ Turn your body to the left, with the right palm turning inwards and the left hand moving back and upwards and both palms facing each other diagonally.

❻ Bringing your left hand near your ear and your right hand back slightly, begin to lift up your right foot.

❼ Step back with your right foot, pushing your left hand forward and pulling the right hand back, while putting all your weight on the right foot. This completes the second Repulse the Monkey.

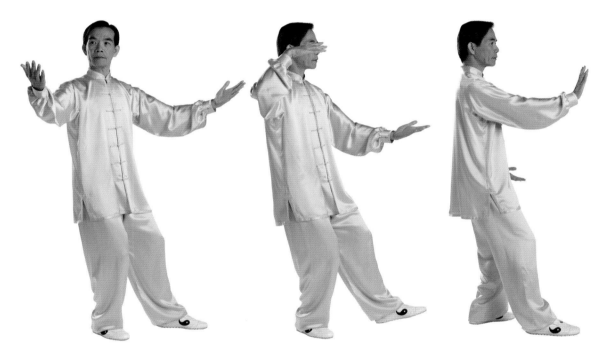

⑧ Turn your body towards the right, right hand moving back and upwards, left palm continuing to turn in, ending with both palms at the same height, facing each other diagonally.

⑨ Bringing your right hand near your ear and your left hand back slightly, begin to lift up your left foot.

⑩ Step back with your left foot, pushing your right hand forward and pulling the left hand backwards, while putting all your weight on the left foot. This completes the third Repulse the Monkey.

The Tai Chi Beginner's Set

REPULSE THE MONKEY

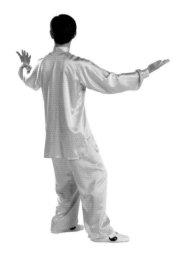

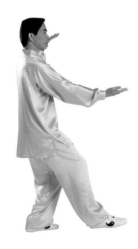

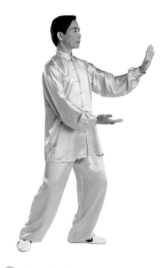

⑪ Turn your body to the left, with the right palm turning inwards and the left hand moving back and upwards.

⑫ Bringing your left hand near your ear and your right hand back slightly, begin to lift up your right foot.

⑬ Step back with your right foot, this time turning the right heel inwards while pushing your left hand forward and pulling the right hand back. This completes the fourth Repulse the Monkey.

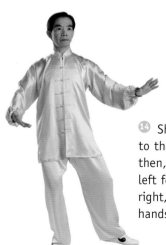

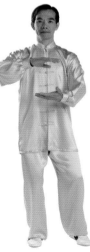

⑭ Shift the weight to the right foot, then, bringing the left foot near the right, bring both hands around.

⑮ Continue to move the hands, moving the right hand up and the left hand down as if you are carrying a ball.

Movement 7
CLOSING

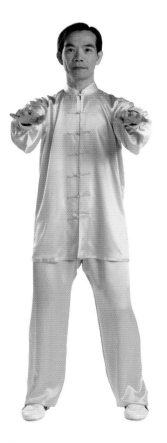

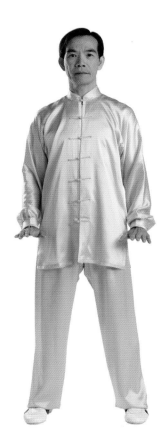

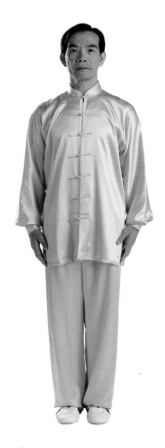

① Place your left foot so that both feet are parallel and shoulder-width apart. Stretch both hands out in front, palms down.

② Press your hands down and slowly straighten up.

③ Bring your feet back together.

CHAPTER 4

WHAT'S NEXT?

Remember at the very beginning we explained how we'd feed you information gradually rather than throw it at you all at once? We said we'd present material to you in steps or stages. Well, now's the time to go further, to the next step—if you want to.

Let's assume you have learned the Six Easy Steps. By now, you've probably got the rhythm and feel of tai chi and feel healthier and perhaps enjoy life more. And, chances are, you want to progress further. If so, you have three options: keep practising what you have learned, study the Six Easy Steps in more depth, or move on to more advanced movements.

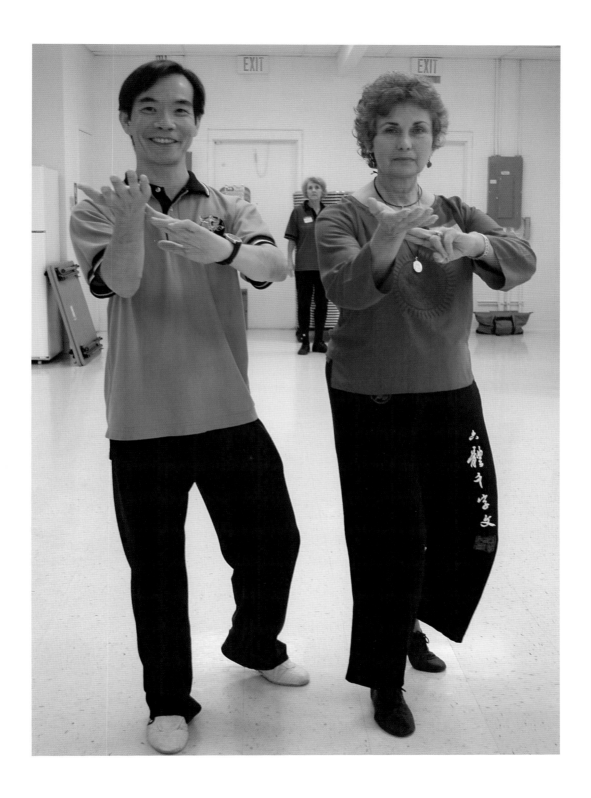

We suggest you continue to practise the original steps for as long as you like or until you have a good handle on them. If your objective in learning tai chi is better health, it's fine to just stick with and keep practising these movements. On the other hand, you might want to tackle something more demanding. The most popular set of tai chi moves is the 24 Forms and that is covered in more detail in Part 2 (see p. 115).

But before you move on, you should consider taking some time to examine the Six Easy Steps more closely. No matter how simple the forms may appear, tai chi has many layers of depth—a bit like the layers within an onion—and as you discover these layers, you'll find yourself enjoying your practice more and gaining more benefits. This chapter will help you do that. Not only will it be challenging, it will help you reach a higher level of tai chi.

As a beginner, you might find some of the concepts in this chapter obscure. If so, don't worry. Just leave whatever you don't understand and move on, keep practising what you do understand and, when appropriate, discuss these ideas with a teacher. As your skills and knowledge improve, you'll find that the concepts will take on somewhat different meanings and begin to make more sense to you. So it's worth revisiting them every now and then.

For the purpose of exploring the steps in more depth, the information in this chapter has been grouped into three sections:
1 Exploring steps 1 and 2
2 Exploring qigong
3 Essential tai chi principles

THE DAN TIAN BREATHING METHOD

This breathing method is a modification of traditional qigong based on modern medical research into the deep stabilizer muscles. It helps to sink your qi to the dan tian and to enhance qi power, which in turn helps improve internal energy. It can be incorporated into all qigong movements. The Heaven and Earth stretch (see p. 40 and p. 103) is a good movement for practising this. Before you start, make sure you are familiar with the abdominal breathing method described on p. 55.

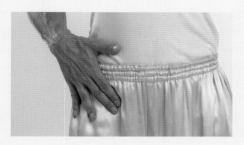

You can practise the breathing either sitting or standing upright. Be aware of holding the correct upright and supple posture. Put one hand on your abdomen just above the belly button and one hand beside your hip with your index and middle fingers just above the groin as shown in the picture.

◼ Concentrate on your lower abdomen and the pelvic floor muscles.

◼ When you inhale, expand your lower abdominal area—allow it to bulge out a little—and let your muscles relax. As you exhale, gently contract the pelvic floor muscles and the lower abdomen. Feel the contraction of the muscles with the index and middle fingers of your right hand, keeping the area above your belly button still. Contract the pelvic floor muscles gently, so gently that it's almost like you're just thinking about it. Alternatively, imagine that you're bringing your pelvic floor a centimetre closer to your belly button. A stronger contraction would move the area above your belly button, which would use a different group of muscles and not be as effective.

◼ As you inhale and release the pelvic and lower abdominal muscles, try not to relax them completely but retain approximately 10–20 per cent of the contraction.

◼ During the Heaven and Earth stretch, inhale as your hands come closer (as though you are carrying a ball). As you move your hands apart (up and down), exhale with your lower abdomen contracting. You'll find the upper limbs move appropriately with your breathing, assisting the correct execution of the dan tian breathing.

We worked with many tai chi and exercise colleagues to create the following deeper versions of the first two steps. Initially, don't worry about the tai chi principles involved. Incorporate them later on when you become more familiar with the sequence. See also pp. 34–5.

Step 1

Warm-up

Walking around sounds simple enough. But you can apply tai chi principles to make it more rewarding. For example:

* Be aware of your posture; be upright, supple and not tense. Imagine your torso is a string and you are gently stretching it from both ends. The top of the string is the midpoint of your head (an acupuncture or energy point called *Bai Hui*) and the bottom of the string is the point between the anus and sexual organ (*Hui Yin*).

* Be aware of your balance and your transference of weight. Focus on centring yourself. Place your weight on one leg. Then adjust your balance and align your body. Lift the other leg up, just above ground, not too high because it will weaken your balance. Take a step within your comfort zone. Touch down lightly with your heel, like a cat, and then gradually transfer your weight forward, in an upright, well-balanced posture. Repeat this with each step, slowly and evenly.

* Be aware of your breathing. It should be gentle and slow.

Step 2

Stretching

See also pp. 36–47

NECK
HEAD DOWN

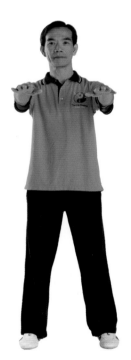

❶ Inhale, loosening your body, and maintaining the right posture. Slowly bring your hands and arms up from your shoulders as though balloons are tied to your wrists. Allow them to float up, but at the same time imagine a gentle resistance against your hands. This will train you to use inner force when moving rather than just lifting your hands without thinking, as you do many times each day.

As you lift your hands, gently push your shoulders downwards. This will allow your shoulders to loosen, enhancing your flow of qi. With practice, you should feel more qi in your palms as you raise them.

TURNING HEAD

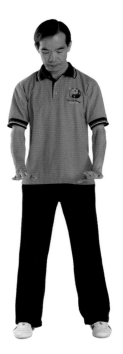

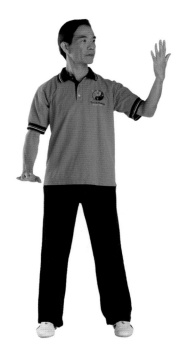

2 When you push your hands forward, exhale and imagine that you're pushing against a gentle resistance. At the same time, imagine an opposing force extending in the opposite direction from your hands to the area between the shoulder blades. Your hands and back will then be stretching in opposite directions, which will help loosen the joints. (Classic tai chi texts refer to this as "force going through to the back".) Still exhaling, bring your hands and arms down, allowing your qi to sink to the dan tian.

Exhale slowly as you look at your palm and gently turn your head to the left. At the same time, gently stretch your shoulder outwards from within. Maintain a small space in your armpit. Your elbow should be bent slightly, pointing diagonally downwards. Gently stretch it downwards. At the same time, imagine stretching your middle finger upwards in the opposite direction. Often referred to as "sinking your elbow", this stretches the tendons and muscles, in turn improving flexibility and enhancing the flow of qi.

Stretching

SHOULDERS
SHOULDER ROLL

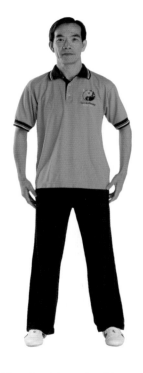

GATHERING QI

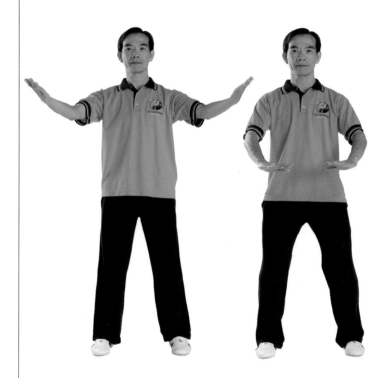

The shoulders should be down, loosened and comfortable. Breathing naturally, be sure the rolling is gentle, circular and continuous, like the classic fluid motions of tai chi.

❶ Inhaling, bring your hands up, imagining that you're gathering qi energy from the universe while stretching your upper limbs. Gently expand from within all the joints of the upper limbs. Loosening all joints, an essential principle of tai chi, enhances qi flow and improves the strength of all ligaments and joints.

❷ As you exhale and slowly bring your hands down, direct your qi down towards the dan tian. If you don't know how to direct your qi down, just think of the dan tian area as you move, and, most likely, in time, it will come to you.

SPINE
HEAVEN AND EARTH

SPINE TURN

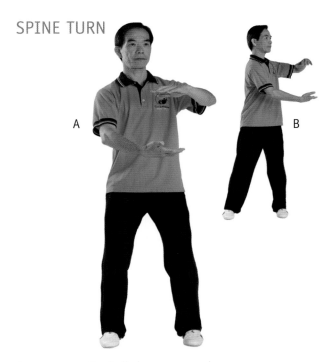

A   B

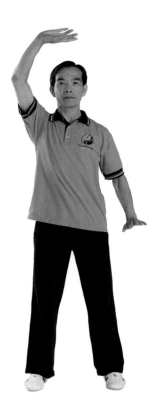

Exhale as your hands stretch up and down. As you stretch, imagine your spine is a string, being stretched gently from both ends. Visualize each vertebra opening up, one by one.

To get the most out of this stretch, combine it with dan tian breathing (see p. 99).

As you carry the ball, be sure your knees are slightly bent. Use your waist to direct the movement as you turn to the side. At the same time, breathe out and sink your qi to the dan tian (or imagine you're doing it). Visualize that the internal power of your waist is transferred to your hands, as if you are moving against resistance. Keep your back upright and joints loosened, turning no more than 45 degrees from the centre so as not to interrupt your qi or strain your posture.

Photo A shows the right way to do this and B the wrong way. Notice that the right way has the hands placed in a vertical line between them and the knee. Avoid turning too much: it can cause excessive strain to the back.

Stretching

HIPS
FORWARD STRETCH

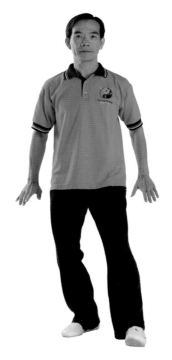

Keep your movements slow, even and continuous. Practise maintaining an upright, balanced posture with flowing movements—like water flowing smoothly in a river. Practise loosening your hip by imagining that your crouched legs form a curved shape like an arch and that you are gently expanding your hip joint. Check yourself in the mirror. Be sure you're mobilizing the qi and stretching the hip joints from within.

SIDE STRETCH

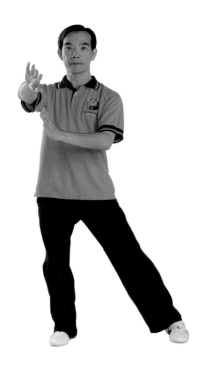

Imagine there's a wall by your side, about an arm's length away. Turn both your palms so that they're pushing against the wall, fingertips forward. At the same time, extend the other foot to the side. Stretching out sideways and keeping the arched shape of your crouched legs in mind, maintain your balance as you push, and sink your qi. Loosen your hip and knee joints. Imagine your torso is the axis, with your upper and lower limbs stretching out in opposite directions. Centring the torso while stretching out in the opposite direction improves your balance and strengthens your qi.

KNEES
KICK

Maintain the correct body posture as you kick and punch out.

As you punch, focus on transferring the force from your dan tian to your hands. Bend your supporting knee slightly for more stability, and stay supple as you kick out. This exercise will train you to focus your mind on how to deliver internal force and at the same time build strength in your legs.

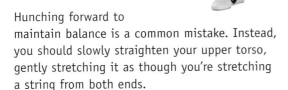

Hunching forward to maintain balance is a common mistake. Instead, you should slowly straighten your upper torso, gently stretching it as though you're stretching a string from both ends.

Make sure you punch with internal force, which is a gentle force originating in the dan tian. If you're not familiar with internal force, you can focus on moving the fist forward as though moving against an imagined gentle resistance. Avoid using brutal force like a karate punch. Eventually the internal force will come to you. When you've loosened your joints, corrected your posture, and learned to use the dan tian breathing method to exhale as you punch, you'll eventually feel the power of the qi. And as you practise this exercise, your balance and strength will improve.

STEP FORWARD

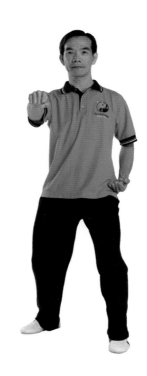

Step forward and focus on the correct stance. Be aware of transferring your weight forward, slowly and gradually. Your internal force (or intention) starts from the back foot, goes to the waist (dan tian), spine, shoulder and arm, and finally expresses itself through the fist. At the same time, be aware of the other fist, for yin and yang balance. (The punch fist is yang, the other is yin. They need to be in balance with each other.)

Exploring qigong

Remember Joanne in Chapter 1? She said, after doing tai chi for eight years, "Physically, I can handle stress a lot better than I used to … I find that overall I handle people and stressful situations differently."

What she was talking about was balance—the key to health. And that's where qigong comes in. Qigong is a form of concentrated practice for better balance of the self. Yes, some form of stress is good for us because it stimulates us and provides a balance for relaxation. Nature goes in circles. Fast complements slow. Full moon alternates with no moon. It's in our nature to be stressed and relaxed, depressed and happy, moving fast and slow—as long as appropriate balance is achieved. Too much stress causes anxiety, but without stress there is no meaning for relaxation.

The great technological advances of the last two hundred years have changed our society. They've changed our relationship with nature, with other human beings and with our own inner selves. Tai chi qigong helps to bring back part of what we've lost, so that we function better in today's world.

Mind-related problems have been conservatively estimated to constitute more than half of the root causes of medical consultations. The main mind-related problems are anxiety (from excess stress) and depression. In Western medicine, we tend to think that these are caused by society

(including interpersonal relationships) and by chemical imbalances in the brain. In traditional Chinese medicine, these conditions are thought to be caused by an imbalance of qi.

In Western medicine, most kinds of exercise have been found to provide relief of stress and depression. Traditional Chinese medicine more specifically prescribes a mind–body exercise such as tai chi qigong. It is reasonable to assume that such mind–body exercises are even more effective in the relief of mind-related problems, and we are sure studies will prove this in time.

Getting into qigong

Qigong exercises may appear simple. They're not. Yes, they are easy to learn, but once you have learned them, their infinite depth and the powerful effect they have on health, especially mental health, will become clear to you with regular practice. And remember, you can practise them almost anywhere and at any time.

Take, for example, the first posture in the qigong exercises, the Posture of Infinity (see p. 51). This posture can be incorporated into anything you do. When you walk, sit, sleep and especially when you practise tai chi, you can be aware of correct posture and your presence in space. And as you practise this seemingly simple posture, you will become aware of its depth.

Gradually, if you allow your body to loosen, your qi to sink, and incorporate essential principles (see p. 112) in your exercises, you'll be able to mobilize and enhance your qi wherever you are.

Let's suppose you're stressed. If you apply the principles of body awareness, sinking the qi, and use dan tian breathing (see p. 99), most likely you'll become more serene and more energized. And the more you've practised and the higher the level you've reached, the easier it will be for you to snap into this meditative state, in which you can focus and be fully aware of the present, but still be serene.

In all Chinese internal martial art styles, qi is the driving force of the internal power (*jin*). The mind (*yi*) directs the qi. Qigong, the exercise of qi cultivation, is an integral part of tai chi. By concentrating on qi cultivation, you can enhance your internal power. High-level tai chi practitioners have great internal power. This power is not necessarily the same as Bruce Lee's—it shows as much in their mental strength as well as in their physical ability.

The qigong exercises in Chapter 3, Step 4 (see p. 50), include techniques to feel the qi and circulate it. (If you have not done or have forgotten Step 4, please go back and review it before proceeding, otherwise the rest of this section may not make sense to you.) It doesn't matter how long it takes you to feel the qi. Every minute you've spent on the exercises will help you gain worthwhile health benefits. Your qi will improve with practice (whether you feel it or not), and as your qi improves, it will automatically integrate into your tai chi and give it more internal power. Qi can be like an elusive lady (or man): when you try too hard to find her (or him), she (or he) will not be there. The key is to practise qigong or tai chi regularly and correctly; then the qi feeling will come to you.

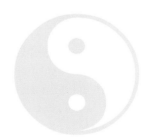

The following two concepts will enhance your qigong practice.

Opening and closing

Opening and closing movements are present in all styles of tai chi. Imagine drawing a bow and shooting an arrow. The drawing is opening and storing energy; the shooting is closing and releasing energy. Keep these mental images in mind because they'll be useful later. We use them frequently when practising tai chi.

In qigong, correct breathing is vitally important. The fundamental concept is: inhale while "drawing the bow" and exhale while "shooting the arrow". For example, at the beginning of Parting the Wild Horse's Mane (see p. 62), when you're carrying the ball, you breathe in to store energy; when you separate your palms to deliver force, you breathe out, since this is a closing movement (even though outwardly it appears to be opening the arms). When you are inhaling, qi moves upwards; when you are exhaling, qi sinks downwards—as in the Posture of Yin-Yang Harmony (see p. 56).

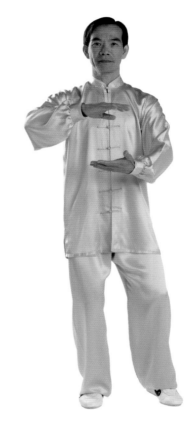

Opening is often described as stretching out. It's important to be aware that the muscles, ligaments, and tendons can be stretching out internally even while you're bringing your limbs closer to your body. When stretching out, be sure not to stretch to the extent of becoming stiff. That will stop your flow of qi. The converse is true when it comes to relaxing. Collapsing all your muscles completely will give you no strength. When you're stretching out, imagine a gentle internal expansion of the joints, muscles and ligaments from within. Apply this to your tai chi forms. Similarly, you should never open (extend) your joints fully, to the extent of locking them, because it will impede the qi flow.

Opening and closing, breathing in and breathing out, all in an alternating pattern—that's the law of nature, and of all tai chi movements. Tai chi uses circular movements to facilitate the circulation of qi, and to make the transfer of energy smooth and continuous. Internal energy becomes stronger as it flows continuously, all the while gathering more qi. This is better illustrated by the next concept.

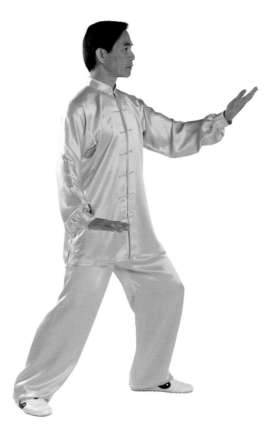

The circulation of qi

To many people, the goal of tai chi is "to live forever and to stay forever young", and according to traditional Chinese medicine the key to health and longevity is qi. Though no-one lives forever, more and more scientific evidence shows that tai chi promotes health and longevity.

When we're born, we're given abundant "essential qi"—have you noticed how lively the very young are? As we grow older, however, our natural qi deteriorates—unless we do something about it. That "something" can be all the components of healthy living, such as exercise, good food and an active lifestyle. Tai chi is one of the most powerful "somethings" that will enhance your qi.

Qigong and tai chi are designed to retain and cultivate qi. Learning to be aware of your qi will help you direct its circulation. According to traditional Chinese medicine, qi moves upwards and continuously escapes from the body through the top of the head (the Bai Hui point). Qigong circulates qi so that it is retained and enhanced.

Once you understand the opening and closing concept, the next stage is to move the qi upwards along the torso as you breathe in. Breathe with your mouth gently closed and your tongue lightly touching the upper palate (roof of the mouth), while you take the qi to the middle of your chest

between both nipples, the acupuncture point known as Shan Zhong.

As you exhale, bring your qi down to the dan tian. Avoid forced breathing. If you run out of breath or are not sure what comes next, then allow yourself to breathe naturally. Eventually, when the body posture and the movements are correct, the right breathing will come naturally.

It might take a long time before you can move the qi as we've described above. Among other things, it depends on your health, and the frequency of practice. Usually, when your tai chi movements are well balanced, when their flow is even and strong, and when your postures are correct, you'll start feeling your qi. Even if you cannot feel your qi, you can still work on circulating qi by visualizing.

After a period of time, and when you are able to feel the qi move this way, you can then process to a higher stage: to circulate your qi through the two major acupuncture meridians or "energy channels".

These energy channels are called the "governing vessel" and the "conception vessel". The governing vessel starts from the acupuncture point Hui Yin, a midpoint between the anus and the sexual organ. It is a narrow channel that travels from this point upwards just underneath the skin and along the midline of the back of the body up to the Bai Hui point—a point on the top and centre of the head. The conception vessel starts from Bai Hui and travels downwards just underneath the skin and along the midline of the front of the body to the Hui Yin point. Thus, the two channels join to form a continuous loop.

As you inhale, picture yourself moving your qi, or internal energy, along the governing vessel, and as you exhale, move your energy down along the conception vessel. With continuous breathing, your energy moves along in this loop, which is also known as microcosmic circulation. The path of the loop is called microcosmic orbit. Again, it doesn't matter if you can't move your energy this way. Simply visualizing or thinking about the path as you breathe will benefit you and improve your tai chi.

It's important not to force the breathing or the qi. Whenever you experience any discomfort or difficulty, simply relax and breathe naturally and stop trying to drive qi. Like nature, when the time is right, your breathing and qi will come together.

To sum up, strong qi does more than improve your tai chi. It also makes you healthier. But is practising qigong enough? No. If you practise qigong without the flowing movements of tai chi, you won't learn the tai chi skills of integrating the internal and external. Moving and exercising

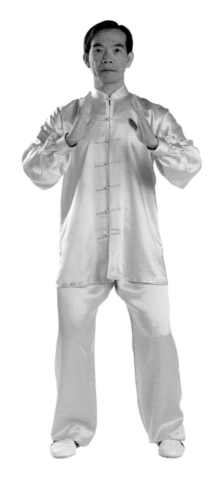

all parts of the body improves flexibility, muscular strength and general fitness. A system that combines both approaches—moving the entire external body and cultivating qi internally—will improve health and skills far more effectively than practising qigong alone.

Essential tai chi principles

Tai chi is a sophisticated art with many different styles and forms. Despite the many variations of tai chi, its immense power for improving health and inner energy derives from a set of essential principles.

Here we present the most important ones. We've put them into simple, easy-to-understand language. By bearing them in mind as you learn and practise, you'll be able to do tai chi more effectively right from the beginning. To see if you're following these principles, you can use a video camera or a mirror, or check with a friend or instructor.

1 Do your movements slowly, without stopping. Make them smooth and continuous like water flowing in a river. Don't jerk. Maintain the same speed throughout.

2 Imagine you're always moving against resistance. That will cultivate your inner force (qi). Imagine the air around you is becoming denser and that every move you make is against a gentle force—as when you move in water.

3 Be conscious of weight transference. This is important for improving mobility, coordination and stability. Be aware when you shift your weight and be aware of each step of your weight transference. When you move forward, for example, put your weight on one leg while maintaining an upright posture. With the upper body vertical to the floor, touch down gently with the other heel first, and then place the entire foot on the ground by gradually shifting your weight onto that foot.

4 Maintain an upright posture and body alignment. Keeping the body straight, without creating tension, is important and can be more difficult than you might expect, especially when you start bending your knees. Very often, when people bend their knees the body alignment becomes distorted.

Test yourself by standing side-on to a mirror. Don't look at the mirror until after you have bent your knees. Now, is your upper body vertical? A good way to maintain good alignment as you do this is to imagine you're going to sit on an empty chair. Bend both your knees and your hip joints. Practise this with the mirror and check yourself every now and then. Once you have achieved good body alignment, your tai chi will improve greatly because qi flows best in a well-aligned body. Hunching forward will hinder the qi flow and compromise your balance, and leaning backwards will impede qi flow and

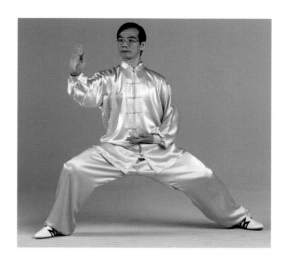

create extra strain on the spine. So try to keep your body upright throughout all movements.

5 Loosen or "song" the joints. You should relax when you do tai chi, but by relax we don't mean let your muscles get floppy. Instead, consciously and gently stretch your joints from within, almost like you're expanding your joints internally. Many people mis-translate the Chinese word *song* as just "relaxation", which is wrong. "Song" means "relaxed and loosened".

To practise loosening the upper limbs, form a semicircle with your arms in front of your chest and imagine all your joints are stretching out gently from within. If you stretch out your shoulder joint this way, you should see a dimple at the middle of the shoulder joint (see below).

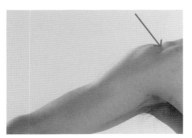

To loosen the spine, imagine it's a string, and that you're gently stretching it from both ends. For the lower limbs, bend your knees, crouch and stretch your hips out to form an arch with your thighs (as shown in this movement). Other lower limb joints will gently expand from within.

6 Focus on your movements. Avoid distraction. Concentrate on what you're doing. Be aware of all the principles mentioned above, but think of them one at a time.

Another set of tai chi

Now you can go back to Step 2 and join all the movements together. Use your creativity to make up some slow and circular linking movements that allow you to flow smoothly from each of the main movements to the next. Then incorporate all of the above principles and you will have learned a new tai chi set.

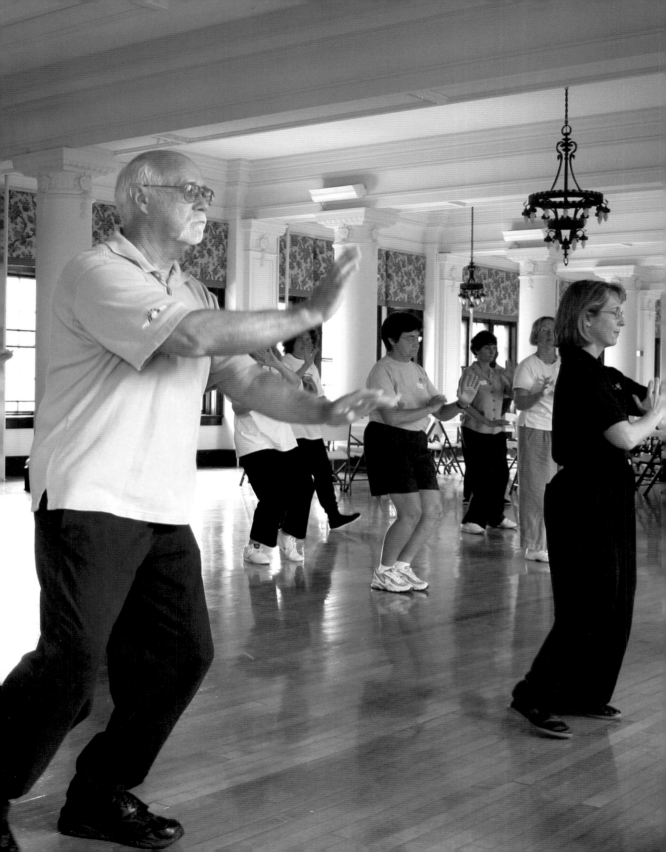

PART 2

THE
24 FORMS

CHAPTER 5

WHAT YOU WANT TO KNOW ABOUT TAI CHI

Over the past 20 years Dr Lam has given numerous talks, conducted workshops and interacted with many thousands of people. Nancy, too, has taught tai chi to novices as well as advanced practitioners and tai chi teachers. Our students come from a wide range of backgrounds—doctors, lawyers, office workers, factory workers, people with different disabilities and chronic conditions, children, young adults—and they've asked all kinds of questions about tai chi. In the following chapter, we've based our information on their questions—assuming you would want to know the same.

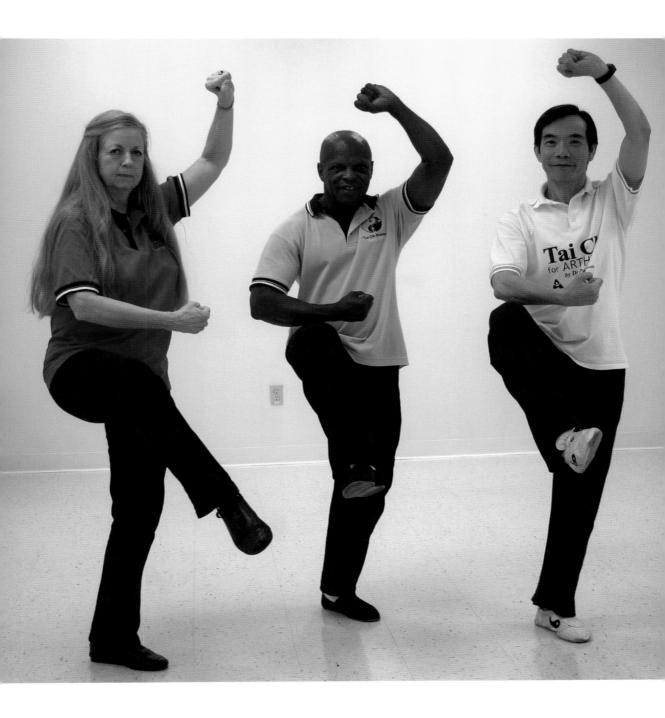

What is tai chi? How does it improve health? How can I learn it? These are the three most common questions that we're asked about tai chi. We've covered the health benefits in Chapter 1, and the bulk of our book is about how to learn tai chi. In this chapter, we address the first question—What is tai chi?—as well as other related questions.

What is tai chi?

Responses to this question might range from "It's a gentle, beautiful exercise that people do in the park" to "It's a martial art" and "It's exercise that people do to improve their health."

Which is right? They all are. Yet, there's much more to tai chi, and virtually no-one can describe such a complex art in one simple sentence. Yes, it's aesthetically pleasing, and most people practising tai chi enjoy themselves. Certainly, it's a most effective martial art. It can also be seen as a form of meditation, a way of fostering the Taoist spirit of living in harmony with nature, of contributing to the preservation of a youthful mind and body. You can call it an art that embraces the mind, the body and the spirit. But as you look over the list of tai chi's attributes, you'll realize they fall under one heading, even under one word: health. The practice of tai chi offers immense health benefits, strengthening both body and mind.

Tai chi can be easy to learn and can become a way of life for practitioners. Yet, because of its depth, no-one ever knows it all, and therein lies part of its fascination and the never-ending challenge of the art.

As you practise tai chi, you'll find, even for the briefest moments, that you'll enter a mental state of complete tranquillity, a world apart, where time and space and the hustle and bustle of life are all left behind. Yet, you'll still feel very much a part of the world. In a non-religious sense, this is a spiritual experience—an experience so satisfying that it's beyond words. It's a mental state expressed by the modern phrase "in the zone"—a state in which you feel totally absorbed and at your personal best. Research shows that the more time a person is "in the zone", the more that person will enjoy life and be fulfilled.

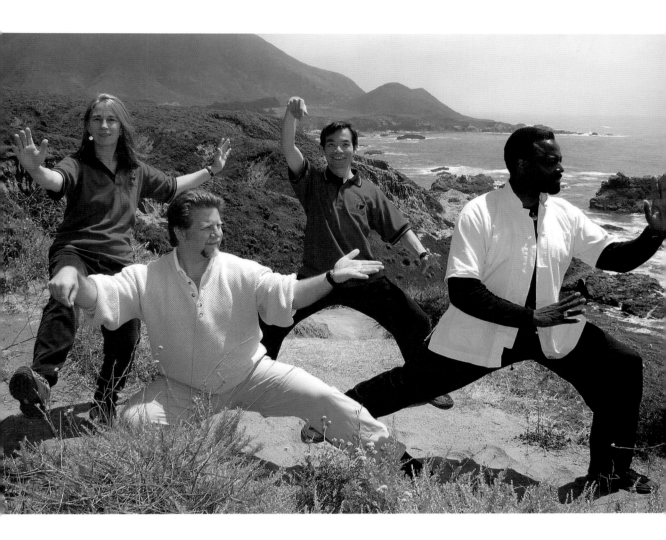

The history of tai chi

Known as *taijiquan* or *tai chi chuan* in China, tai chi is also sometimes called "shadow boxing." It is one of the major branches of the traditional Chinese martial-art form known as *wushu*.

The words tai chi mean "infinity" or "vastness to the absolute extreme" and reflect ancient Chinese concepts of how the universe developed. According to ancient Chinese philosophy, the universe started as a vast void. From this, it developed into a state of tai chi—infinity or vastness to the ultimate extreme.

The word *quan* or *chuan* means "fist". It appears at the end of the names of all Chinese martial-art styles—for example,

---

MASTERS OF TAI CHI

■ **Chen Wang-ting (mid-seventeenth century)**
The creator of tai chi, Chen Wang-ting was a general in the Chinese army. Upon retirement, he was appointed head of his village's army, something akin to being a local commander of an army reserve unit. At the time, however—about 1644—the Ming Dynasty had just been taken over by the Qing Dynasty. Frustrated by his inability to develop his military career, he diverted his excess energy into creating tai chi.

Chen Wang-ting based tai chi on contemporary knowledge of martial arts, in which he was an expert. In Chen-style tai chi, one can see traces of the then-popular martial-art forms, as well as traditional Chinese medicine, qigong and philosophical understanding of nature.

We suspect that from the start, the martial-art element was but one of many facets of tai chi. At the time, however, presenting the activity as a martial art, rather than as an exercise to improve health, was probably the best way to market it.

---

xingyiquan and shaolinquan. *Tai chi chuan* is therefore a martial art based on an understanding of the universe.

The first known written reference to tai chi dates back 3000 years and appeared in the *I Ching* (*The Book of Changes*) during the Zhou Dynasty (1221–1100 BC). In this book, it says, "in all changes exists *taiji*, which causes the two opposites in everything"—a reference to yin and yang. The history of tai chi remains hazy, however. Some accounts attribute its beginnings to a famous fifteenth-century Taoist priest, Zhang Shanfeng. But others claim that Zhang Shanfeng never existed and is a character of folklore.

MASTERS OF TAI CHI

■ **Yang Lu-chan (1799–1872)**
Yang is the style of tai chi most frequently taught in the Western world. It was developed by Yang Lu-chan, who loved martial arts and who had, since his youth, studied with many famous masters. One day, when sparring with a descendant from the Chen village, Yang became fascinated by the amazing power and unusual combination of softness and hardness of his opponent's tai chi. Chen style was not taught to outsiders. But Yang was so eager to learn the art that he pretended to be a starving beggar and fainted at the front door of a Chen village elder; as he had planned, he was then taken in and accepted as a servant in the Chen household.

At night, Yang would peer through a crack in the wall to watch Chen-style tai chi practice, and then practise in secret. After a few years, he became a highly skilled practitioner. But his deception was eventually discovered. In those days, Yang could have been legally executed for such an act, but the Chen clan leader was so impressed with Yang's skill that he took him on as his first non-Chen student.

Yang later travelled around China to teach the art of tai chi. Called "Yang the Invincible," he gained a great reputation. Eventually, he developed his own style, which was more open and gentle than Chen tai chi.

Yang Lu-chan remains an extreme example of how one can become so addicted to tai chi that one is willing to risk one's life to practise it!

Towards the modern era

More reliable accounts come out of the sixteenth century. They attribute the development of tai chi to Chen Wang-ting, a sixteenth-century retired army general of the Chen village in Wenxian County, Henan Province. After he retired from the army, Chen Wang-ting led a simple life of farming but also, under the influence of Taoism, studied and taught martial arts. In the 1670s, he developed several tai chi routines. He was greatly influenced by the martial-arts schools that existed in those days, including that of the famous general of the imperial army, Qi Jiguang, who wrote *Boxing in 32 Forms*, an important textbook on military training.

Perhaps even more significantly, along with Taoists' understanding of nature, Chen Wang-ting incorporated into his martial-art routines the traditional Chinese medicine and qigong exercises. Both techniques later evolved into qigong exercises. By combining the martial arts with qigong, the ancient philosophical understanding of nature, as well as aspects of traditional Chinese

MASTERS OF TAI CHI

■ Sun Lu-tang (1861–1932)

Sun Lu-tang was a famous master of two other internal arts, xingyiquan (a fighting style based on the integration of internal energy and external appearance) and baguaquan (a fighting style based on eight diagrams of the *I-Ching, The Book of Changes*).

One day, Sun happened to meet Hao Wei-zheng, one of the best exponents of tai chi at that time. Hao was sick. Without knowing Hao's identity, Sun, as a good humanitarian, found Hao a hotel room and a good doctor to treat him. When Hao was on the road to recovery, he moved into Sun's house for three months to teach him tai chi. At the time, Sun was over 50 years old, but not only did he learn tai chi, he combined it with his own internal styles—xingyiquan and baguaquan—to create Sun-style tai chi.

History regards Sun as one of the highest achievers of the art of tai chi, and it's interesting to note that he didn't start his training as a child as did many of the other masters. Starting tai chi at a relatively late age and spending only a short period of time learning it, Sun created one of tai chi's most important styles—a perfect example of not being limited by age or lineage. Sun made tai chi accessible to people of all classes and abilities. For example, he was the first to openly teach women, and he wrote the first book on tai chi's health benefits.

medicine, Chen made tai chi a complete system of exercise in which the practitioner's mental concentration, breathing and actions were closely connected.

It's likely that Chen intended his art to be a form of health care. Good health and longevity would no doubt have been on his mind given that he was entering old age. With a view to maintaining his physical and mental wellbeing, he could have been investigating the idea of combining qigong and traditional medicine with a martial art.

Tai chi was passed on to and refined by further generations of the Chen family, but wasn't widely practised outside the area of Chen's village until the early nineteenth century. That's when Yang Lu-chan learned Chen-style tai chi. Yang Lu-chan soon became a highly skilled and enthusiastic practitioner, developing his own particular style of tai chi. The other major styles of tai chi practised today include the two Wu styles, and the Sun style. All of these styles originated directly or indirectly from the Chen style.

MASTERS OF TAI CHI

■ Chen Fa-ke (1887–1957)

A direct descendant of Chen Wang-ting, Chen Fa-ke was sickly and weak as a child. While he was growing up, his father often travelled away from home teaching tai chi. Chen was supposed to be learning too, but didn't. He was either too lazy or just not interested.

By the time he reached the age of 15, however, Chen's physical weakness had become an embarrassment to him. In particular, it bothered him that one of his older cousins was well known and respected as the best tai chi exponent in Chen's peer group. Chen wished he could catch up with his cousin, and one day he decided to do something about it.

Chen used every available minute to practise and after a few years he managed to beat his cousin in a friendly contest. People thought his father had taught him in secret. No-one realized that most of the time his father was away, and that Chen had done all the hard work on his own.

That self-motivation characterized Chen's later life. He was a model of consistent practice and a good example of the incredible power of Chen-style tai chi. According to many stories, he was so effective in martial arts that he was known as "the invincible". Stories describe how other well-known martial artists would last only seconds when sparring with him.

The five major styles

Below we list, in chronological order of origin, the five major styles that are practised today. Just because one comes before another doesn't mean we think it's better. Tai chi is a vast reservoir of knowledge, an accumulation of the work of many dedicated people throughout the centuries. Each style has different characteristics and each is unique and valuable in its own way.

Besides these five, there are other styles, not necessarily better or worse or less effective, but simply not as well known; and within each style there are significant differences between the many schools and branches.

Chen style

Devised in the early twentieth century, when Chen Fa-ke (see p. 123), an expert in the Chen style, started teaching tai chi in Beijing. Stories abound about Chen's amazing prowess and also about his near-perfect disposition. He was well liked by all, making no enemies during the 29 years he lived in Beijing, up until his death in 1957.

Chen style is characterized by an emphasis on spiral force (also called *chan suu jin* or "silk-reeling force") and effective martial application. Slow movements intermix with fast; hard movements are complementary to soft. Chen style is also characterized by explosive power and a low stance. The core power, however, comes from the spiral force, an inner force that travels along a spiral path in three dimensions. The potential application of this style to combat techniques makes it enticing to younger people, but it is difficult to learn.

Yang style

The most popular style today, the Yang style was created in the early nineteenth century by Yang Lu-chan (see p. 121). Yang learned tai chi at the Chen village and later developed his own style, which he taught to a great number of people, including the members of the imperial court.

The movements of the Yang style are gentle, graceful, effective for promoting health, and easier to learn than those of the Chen style. Yang style is suitable for almost all ages and physical conditions. The 24 Forms and the Tai Chi Beginner's Set are based on the Yang style.

Hao style

This style is commonly known in China as the Wu style, though the Chinese name differs from that of the other Wu style (see below). To differentiate the two Wu styles, we will call this one by its other name, Hao.

This style was created by Wu Yu-xiang (1812–80) and passed on to Hao Wei-zheng (1849–1920), who made a significant contribution to the style. It is characterized by close-knit, slow movements. Great emphasis is placed on internal power and correct positioning. Hao is a relatively uncommon style.

Wu style

The other Wu style was created by Wu Jian-quan (1870–1942). It is characterized by softness and emphasis on re-directing incoming force. Its movements are relaxed, nimble and made close to the trunk of the body. The style is rich with hand techniques, especially in "push hands", an exercise practised by two people as a gentle alternative to sparring (see p. 126). The postures in Wu-style tai chi often involve leaning slightly forward.

Sun style

The youngest of the major styles, the Sun style, was created by Sun Lu-tang (see p. 122). It is distinguished by agile steps: whenever one foot moves forward or backwards, the other foot follows. The style's movements flow smoothly like water in a river. Incorporating the essence of two other internal martial arts—xingyiquan and baguaquan—Sun style includes a unique and powerful form of qigong that is especially effective for relaxation and healing. Its higher stance makes it easier and safer for older people to learn and practise.

Dr Lam has created several Tai Chi for Health programs based solely or partly on Sun style. These programs have helped hundreds of thousands of people improve their health and quality of life.

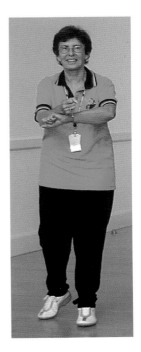

Tai chi as a martial art

Most people practise tai chi for its health benefits. However, tai chi was originally known as a martial art, and there are still many people who practise it as a form of self-defence. Understanding the martial-art aspect of tai chi helps all practitioners do the movements more correctly, build internal energy and concentrate better. Tai chi was created based on the understanding of nature and its relationship to humans. Martial art is only one of the many facets of tai chi.

Keep in mind that if health is your goal in doing tai chi, martial-art training can give you a higher risk of injury. Learning the tai chi principles as we discussed throughout this book will help you improve your level of tai chi no matter what objective you have. If martial-art training is important to you, we recommend going to a class with a teacher who places emphasis on this aspect. The higher level of your tai chi will give you a solid foundation, but it would be beyond the scope of this book to go into this aspect.

Tai chi's focus on training the mind helps practitioners to think clearly and be well balanced mentally. It helps them assess situations before acting, rather than hitting out immediately in anger. The physical aspect of tai chi helps build strong muscles, flexibility, general fitness, a good sense of balance, an ability to transfer weight efficiently and correct posture. This training is just as useful for health improvement as for martial art.

We shall discuss two aspects of tai chi that you may come across in your journey in tai chi.

PUSH HANDS

This is a clever two-person drill in which participants push each other to feel each other's strength and internal force.

In a one-hand Push Hand drill, one person pushes the other with his or her hand on the other person's wrist, while the other person yields and redirects the incoming force. They then change roles. Through pushing and yielding the players experience the incoming force and how to yield, "listen to" or feel the incoming force, and absorb and redirect this force. In a two-hand Push Hand drill, one hand is touching the other person's wrist and the other is on the elbow. Essentially, they are doing the same push and yielding, but with both hands instead of one. This makes the practice more complex.

There are also many other techniques, such as a two-hand moving drill, and different styles of tai chi have different methods of Push Hands—too many to cover in this book. While pushing hands is a useful tool, and it can be a tool to enhance the martial-art aspect of tai chi skill, it is complex and difficult to learn. Be

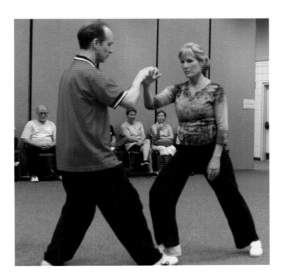

sure to find a teacher who understands your needs and has the right temperament for you. Some teachers place emphasis on the martial-art aspect of Push Hand practice, but there is a higher risk of injury because you cannot predict your opponent's force.

Tai chi competitions

There are now many tai chi competitions around the world. Tai chi is one of the internal martial arts, so is often included as part of a Wu-shu competition. Wu-shu means "Chinese martial art", which is commonly known in the Western world as kung fu. Competitions can be inspirational and fun depending on your approach and attitude. It is certainly a great way to promote tai chi and meet friends.

Most Wu-shu competitions have two components. The first one is a forms competition where competitors perform a set of forms within the time limit and are judged on their competency. The second

TAI CHI CLASSICS

The collections of wisdom from generations of tai chi exponents are often called the "Tai Chi Classics". Some of the older texts were written in classical Chinese; others in more modern Chinese. For example, the *Tai Chi Jing* was written in classical Chinese whereas the *Ten Essential Points* by Yang Chan-fu was written in more modern, but not present-day, Chinese.

If you were to start studying the Tai Chi Classics in English, you would need to be aware of problems inherent in translations. The Chinese language, especially classical Chinese, is artistic and not as precise as English. Also, Chinese words can have a variety of meanings when used for tai chi.

Great treasures exist in the classical texts and, for serious practitioners, exploration of these books can be highly rewarding. Dr Lam has studied the classics in Chinese, and has expressed many of their most important concepts in easy-to-understand language throughout this book.

component is free-style fighting, where there is no specification as to what martial-art style competitors can use. The winner knocks out the loser much the same as boxers in a boxing ring, although the rules and protective gear worn are different.

All competitions have their own specific sets of rules and inclusion criteria. If you are interested in entering competitions, you will need the guidance of a teacher who is interested and familiar with them.

Internal? External? What's it all about?

Hundreds of different martial-art styles come from China. They're broadly divided into two styles: external and internal. The internal stylists place great emphasis on cultivating qi, serenity of the mind, and strengthening the internal structure of the body. They use "soft" strategies, such as yielding, absorbing and redirecting incoming force. They also stress gentleness in combination with self-awareness and breath control. Tai chi, xingyiquan and baguaquan are examples of internal styles.

In contrast, the external schools (also called "hard" schools), such as shaolinquan (similar to karate), place greater emphasis on speed and muscle power. While different external schools have their own philosophies and features, their strategy for combat tends towards blocking, punching and kicking, and matching their opponent with speed and muscle power.

Training with external schools often enables you to use self-defence techniques sooner; in contrast, students who train with internal schools usually take longer to acquire the same self-defence ability. In the long run, however, these students tend to catch up and attain superior skills. Both approaches have their merits; the important thing for the practitioner is to take the time to understand his or her needs and match them to what is offered by a school or teacher.

Many martial artists have learned different martial-art styles. For example, Sun Lu-tang, the creator of the Sun style, was an exponent of both xingyiquan and baguaquan before he learned tai chi. Many practitioners of external martial arts take up tai chi as they get older. The weaker muscles and slower reflexes that come with ageing can be a hindrance in external martial arts, but because tai chi is internal and stresses mind control, the maturity that comes with age is actually an advantage.

The internal components of tai chi

What do we mean when we say "internal"? The word can mean different things. In relation to the body, the mind is internal; the organs are internal to the muscles and the muscles are internal to the skin. We can view this in three ways.

The body

When you are practising tai chi, all the internal organs, joints and ligaments are involved and exercised. Tai chi's unique breathing technique expands the lung capacity, thus improving their function. It also improves your relaxation through the using of abdominal or diaphragmatic breathing (see p. 55).

As you probably know, breathing is closely related to your mental state. For example, when you're excited or nervous, you breathe faster and shallower. When you concentrate on breathing more slowly and more deeply, you become calmer. Deep, slow diaphragmatic breathing, as taught in tai chi, creates alternating pressure in the chest cavity, which gently massages the heart. It opens more air space that is normally unused within the lung, thus increasing the total lung capacity. Deep breathing also exerts pressure on the abdominal cavity, massaging the organs therein.

The mind

The way tai chi integrates mind and body is unique and powerful. In our fast-paced society, as we grow in age we lose more of the connection between the conscious mind and the body.

Check yourself in a mirror or watch yourself on a video. You'll find that your body isn't always doing what you think it is doing. For instance, bend your knees and check yourself. You might think your back is upright, but the mirror may tell you it isn't.

Training your mind so that what your brain thinks, your body does, can help bring you back to nature and harmony. Then, when, for example, you are worried about something, you can tell your body to relax and stop the sweating and fast heartbeat—and it will!

The spirit

The spirit is controlled largely by the unconscious mind. You might be able to consciously make yourself less anxious for a short time, but then you automatically revert to your anxious state because the unconscious mind takes over.

We have found that, to a certain extent, we can use our conscious mind in combination with body training to control the unconscious. For example, using visualization and relaxation techniques, sports psychologists can help athletes to overcome performance anxiety.

In a similar way, tai chi uses visualization techniques to cultivate qi. If done regularly, this can reach the unconscious mind, making it more serene and more positive.

More on qigong

Qigong is an ancient Chinese practice that enhances health and relaxation. Yes, tai chi does that, too. But tai chi differs from qigong in the sense that qigong is a training to cultivate qi, whereas tai chi is a martial art or exercise that incorporates qigong as its core strength.

Qi is the life energy within a person; indeed, according to traditional Chinese medicine, qi is life. It flows through specific channels, called energy channels or meridians—the same meridians as an acupuncturist uses (acupuncture is based on the same concept of qi.) Qi performs many functions such as moving the blood, lymphatic fluid and energy around the body.

A person with strong qi will be healthy and live a long life. Each of us is endowed at birth with essential qi. That essential qi combines with the qi absorbed in the digestive system from food and water and the qi extracted from the air you breathe to form the vital qi of the body. The storage house of qi is the dan tian, an area situated three fingerwidths below the belly button.

The concept of qi is fundamental to traditional Chinese medicine. Practitioners believe that personal qi is related to the qi of the environment and the universe. Qi becomes stronger when you're in harmony with your environment, when you exercise and practise good nutrition and when you enjoy mental tranquillity.

Although numerous forms of qigong exist, it is essentially the practice of cultivating qi. It consists of special breathing exercises and meditation, sometimes integrated with movement. Tai chi incorporates qigong as an integral part of its practice; indeed, the internal power of tai chi for both health and martial-art purposes is the qi. (See pp. 50–57 for qigong exercises and pp. 106–111 for information on how to explore the depth of qigong.)

When you practise qigong exercises without complex movements, you can focus on your inner self, without having to think about moving your arms or legs. This concentration on mental imaging and relaxation will improve your tai chi. Then, you can take that mental stage you reached from qigong practice, and bring it to the fore as you practise your tai chi movements. This will facilitate incorporating qi into the movements and in turn lead to easier body–mind integration.

The most common types of qigong are meditative and breathing exercises. We believe, however, that while meditative exercises are useful, they're not complete as an exercise. An ideal exercise should involve training of the entire body and the mind— as tai chi does.

Tai chi breathing

Correct breathing is an important part of tai chi. It's the basis of gathering, storing and delivering energy, which play a vital part in every tai chi movement. The Tai Chi Classics describe breathing as opening and closing. When you open, you're storing energy, just as when you draw an arrow in a bow; when you close, you're delivering energy, just as when you release and fire the arrow. Keeping this image in mind will help you breathe correctly.

When you're inhaling (storing energy), think of taking life-energy into your body. When you exhale, think of delivering energy or force. This can be applied to all tai chi movements since all movements in all types of tai chi are, in essence, alternating opening and closing movements.

For example, when your hands pull apart or when you're stepping forward, that's an opening movement. In Parting the Wild Horse's Mane (see p. 62), when you place your hands one above the other as if you are carrying a ball, this is when you are storing your energy. Then, when you separate your hands, there's an out-breath and you're delivering energy.

Up-and-down movements fit the same pattern. When you move your hands up, you're storing energy, and therefore you breathe in. When you bring your hands down, you're delivering energy—shooting the arrow—so you breathe out. Likewise when you stand up (breathe in) and bend down (breathe out).

Keep these images in mind whenever you're practising tai chi. When in doubt, focus on practising the form correctly: relax, loosen your joints and you'll find your breathing will most likely be correct. Don't force or hold your breath. Simply allow your body to breathe naturally.

CHAPTER 6

THE 24, 48, 42 AND OTHER SETS OF FORMS

Most styles of tai chi have sets of forms that have been created and passed on through the generations as their core curriculum. This chapter lists the most popular new sets of forms that have been composed and disseminated with different levels of involvement from the Sport Department of the Chinese National Government. These forms are often called official sets of forms, or Beijing New Forms. For each set, we provide some background information and a description of the forms.

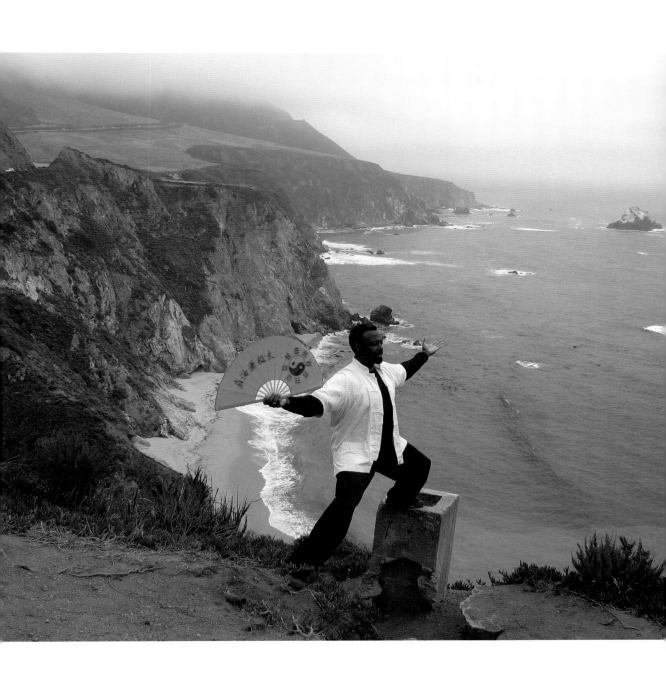

A style? A form? A set? You might ask, "What's the difference between these?" Good question. On p. 124–5, we discussed the five major styles. Almost 99 per cent of today's tai chi belongs to or is a variation of one of those styles.

A "form" is a group of movements that fit into that group for a particular purpose or sequence of purposes. Take Repulse the Monkey, for example: the few movements in that form are designed to cultivate internal energy and also have several martial-art applications. Confusingly, many people also call an entire form a "movement".

A "set" is a sequence of tai chi forms (or movements). In other words, when you string forms together, you create a set, such as the seven forms in the Tai Chi Beginner's Set or the 24 Forms that we'll show you in the next chapter.

With the passing of time, sets are lost, modified and created. This might confuse you; on the other hand, you could see it as an advantage: it's better to have too many choices than too few. Remember, though, you don't have to learn many sets of forms to reach high-level tai chi and to gain major health benefits.

Why practise different forms?

You need practise only one set of forms to reach a high level in tai chi. One of the greatest masters, Hong Jun-sheng, specialized in Chen style's classical sets. In fact, most of the great masters like Yang Chan-fu and Sun Lu-tang practised only their own set. But learning more sets is sometimes advantageous. Different sets and styles have their own unique characteristics and points of interest. Learning more sets and even different styles enriches techniques, broadens practitioners' horizons and offers greater challenges and enjoyment. It depends on your own preference and style of learning. Some people prefer to specialize in one set of forms; others would like to benefit from the variations.

Characteristics of a set might suit one person more than another, so it wouldn't hurt you to at least know something about each different set and style. Some traditional sets are excellent, but they're not all good simply because they're older. Then again, some sets might not suit you because of personal constraints. For example, it can take 20–40 minutes to do the classical Yang-style 108 Forms. Add warm-up and cooling-down exercises, and you'd need nearly two hours to practise three repetitions of this set. How many people can afford this amount of time for daily practice? In contrast, the 24 Forms, which contains all the essential principles

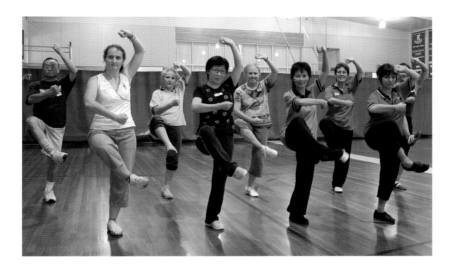

of tai chi, takes only 5 or 6 minutes to complete. Most people find it easier to fit this set into their lives.

Understanding what's in a set

When starting to learn a set of forms, it helps to understand its structure and background. It's like an artist playing a musical composition. Understanding the inner meaning of the composition, the composer's intention and the structure of the piece will be helpful to the artist. So try to find out as much as possible about a set before learning it, because you might spend the rest of your life practising it, and the small amount of time invested in knowing what it's all about will be well worth it.

Sets of forms arranged in specific sequences were put together to facilitate practice and qi cultivation. The construction of these sets was based on essential tai chi principles. A set would start from a spot and return to the same spot, reflecting the way in which nature, working in cycles, returns to where it begins, as reflected in the saying "ashes to ashes" (and also in the yin-yang symbol). A well-constructed set starts with slow, gentle, stretching movements to help the practitioner warm up, gradually builds to a crescendo, then slows down (cooling down), in a way that mirrors nature.

Creators of sets also considered the martial-art needs of practitioners, with sets being constructed in a way that would facilitate sparring. Other factors such as qi cultivation, balance and flow were also important considerations.

Through time, old sets have been refined and new sets created. Indeed, the creation of the 24 Forms was so successful that the Chinese National Sports Committee has commissioned experts to create more sets of forms, some of which are covered below.

The 24 Forms

In 1956, in order to popularize tai chi, the Chinese National Sports Committee authorized four renowned tai chi experts to create the 24 Forms. To do this, the experts condensed the long, classical Yang-style set to just 24 forms. This set quickly became the most popular in the world.

The 24 Forms retains the essential principles of tai chi and is easier to learn, remember and practise than the classical Yang-style forms. Moreover, it takes just five minutes to do the entire set; therefore, including warm-up and cooling-down exercises, one can do three sets in only 30 minutes. Many medical studies on the health benefits of tai chi are based on people practising this set or parts of it.

The structure of the 24 Forms

The 24 Forms is divided into four sections. The first section consists of gentle stretching of the upper and lower limbs, which prepares the body for more vigorous movements. For example, Parting the Wild Horse's Mane includes movements that gently stretch the body, while, in the more demanding second section, Stroking the Bird's Tail requires more strenuous stretching and turning of the body.

The third section of the 24 Forms is where the most difficult, such as heel kicks, are executed. At the end, the slower movements, such as Apparent Closing Up, work as winding-down exercises.

The Combined 48 Forms

Created in 1976 by three tai chi experts, this was the first set to combine forms from four major styles, namely Chen, Yang, Wu and Sun. The goal was to condense the best of all the styles into a short set, in the manner of a condensed version of a classic novel. More complex and technically demanding than the 24 Forms, the 48 Forms was created for demonstration and competition purposes. The idea proved to be popular and effective. The set is well balanced, with most movements being done equally on both sides of the body, and it has a perfect tempo, flows smoothly, and is in keeping with essential tai chi principles.

This is the longest of the newer sets, taking about 8–12 minutes to complete.

The Combined 42 Forms

As tai chi became more popular, competitions flourished, especially within China. Originally, each competitor was asked to compose his own set. That resulted in each competitor performing a different set, making it difficult to set standards for judging. So in the late 1980s, the Chinese National Sports Committee decided to standardize competition sets. A set was created for each of the four major styles, along with one extra set combining the features and characteristics of all four. The combined set is called the Combined 42 Forms or the Competition Forms. Today, most major competitions around the world include this set as one of the most important phases of the competition.

This set also has four sections: Section 1 moves quickly to Movement 2: Stroking the Bird's Tail, which displays a technique and style that attract interest and attention, yet still provides a gentle stretching of the upper and lower body.

Section 2 starts with the Sun style's Movement 11: Opening and Closing. Not only is this the most characteristic movement of the Sun style, it also indicates the importance of qigong within the set. Near the end of this section, the first climax appears with Movement 17: Cover with Hand and Punch with Fist, and Movement 18: Parting Wild Horse's Mane, from the more vigorous Chen style.

Section 3 starts with Movement 19: Waving Hands Like Clouds, a slower and easier movement to break up the intensity, then proceeds to more difficult movements. The second climax starts in Section 4 with movements such as Movement 32: Body Thrust with Half Horse Stance. The set then winds down and finishes off with another Movement 40: Stroking the Bird's Tail on the other side.

Other sets

In the late 1980s, four new national competition sets were created by six leading tai chi experts and approved by a group of well-respected tai chi experts. They are the 56 Chen Style, 40 Yang Style, 45 Wu Style and 73 Sun Style.

These sets retain the traditional characteristics, features and techniques of their respective styles. By incorporating high levels of difficulty and meeting competition standards, they also aim to raise the standard of tai chi in competitions.

CHAPTER 7

LEARNING THE 24 FORMS

The 24 Forms is by far the world's most popular set of forms, firstly because of its beauty and flow, but also because it is easier to learn than the traditional sets and takes less time to perform. There are many interpretations of this set. We have adapted the most authentic version, while placing an emphasis on the essential tai chi principles, all of which are covered. The resulting set is ideal for health improvement and for developing tai chi skills.

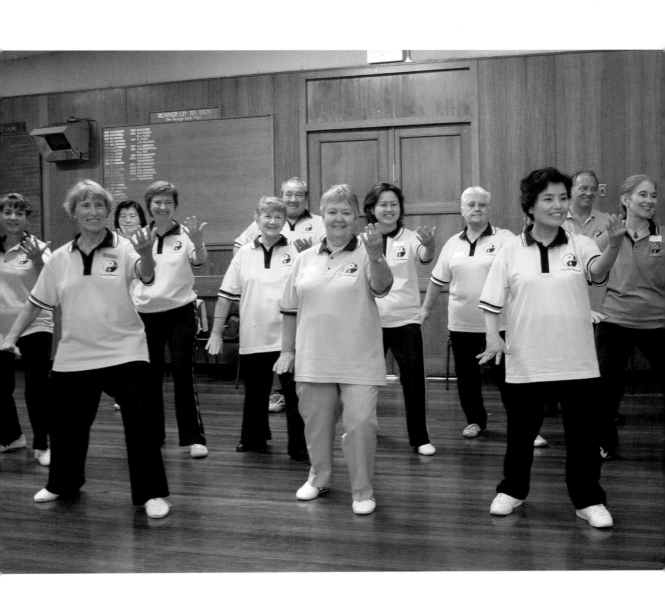

The 24 Forms

Movement 7
STROKING THE BIRD'S TAIL (LEFT)

Because the Tai Chi Beginner's Set is based on the 24 Forms, you'll have no trouble joining them together. At the end of the Beginner's Set, instead of going to the closing movement, continue with Movement 7 of the 24 Forms, Stroking the Bird's Tail.

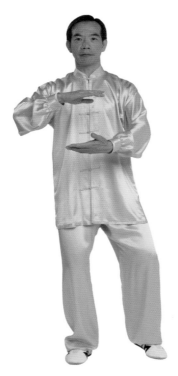

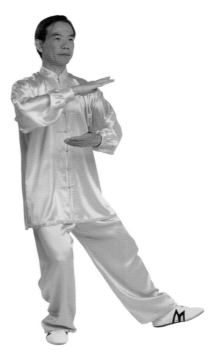

1 Begin where you left off on page 94 (just before "Closing"), with your weight on the right foot, your right hand up and your left hand down as if you are carrying a ball.

2 Step out to the left with your toes pointing to the left. Move the hands inwards slightly, as though you're gently squeezing the ball. This is to initiate the next movement of the hands in the opposite direction.

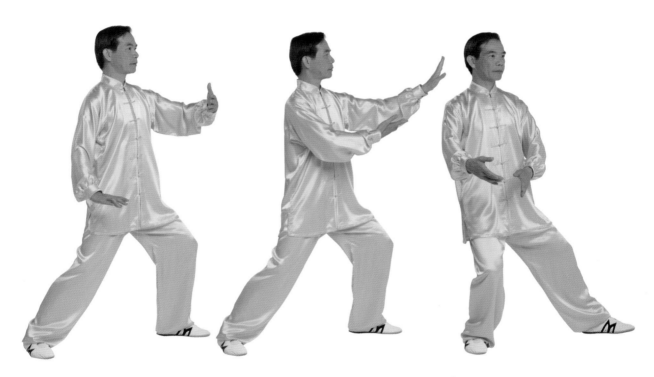

③ Push your left arm forward to form a semicircle in front of your chest and move your right hand next to your hip, with the fingers pointing forward. At the same time, shift your weight forward gradually. This is called Ward Off.

④ Continue to shift your weight forward and, with a slight turn of the waist, turn your left hand out so that the palm is facing diagonally downwards. Turn the right palm up.

⑤ Shift your weight back and bring both arms down and to the right. This is called Roll Back.

The 24 Forms

STROKING THE BIRD'S TAIL (LEFT)

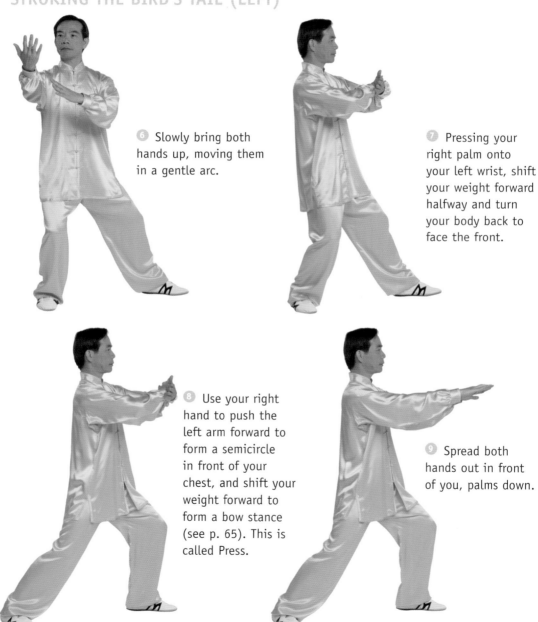

6 Slowly bring both hands up, moving them in a gentle arc.

7 Pressing your right palm onto your left wrist, shift your weight forward halfway and turn your body back to face the front.

8 Use your right hand to push the left arm forward to form a semicircle in front of your chest, and shift your weight forward to form a bow stance (see p. 65). This is called Press.

9 Spread both hands out in front of you, palms down.

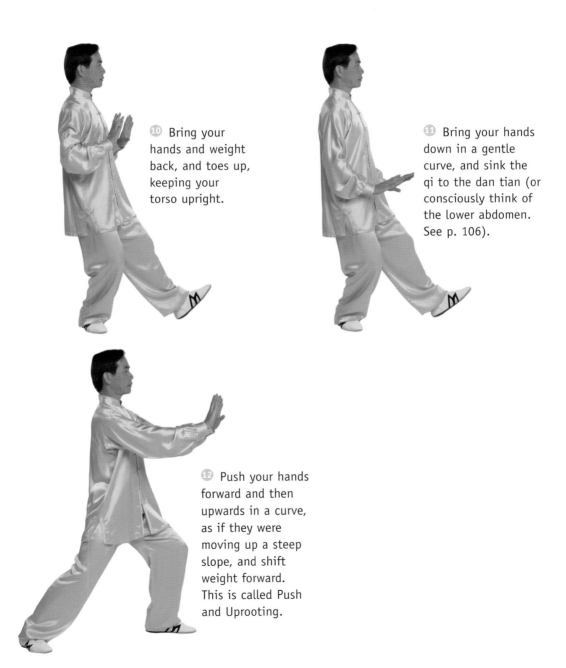

10 Bring your hands and weight back, and toes up, keeping your torso upright.

11 Bring your hands down in a gentle curve, and sink the qi to the dan tian (or consciously think of the lower abdomen. See p. 106).

12 Push your hands forward and then upwards in a curve, as if they were moving up a steep slope, and shift weight forward. This is called Push and Uprooting.

The 24 Forms

Movement 8
STROKING THE BIRD'S TAIL (RIGHT)

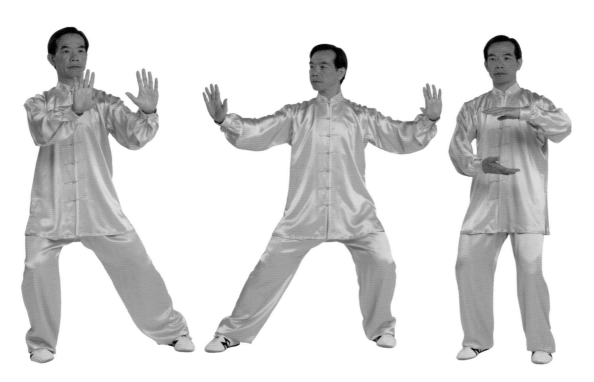

❶ Shift your weight backwards, then turn the left toes inwards to face the front (12 o'clock position).

❷ Turn your right toes outwards to be parallel with the left toes, and open up both arms.

❸ Shift your weight onto the left foot, and bring your arms to the front of the chest as though you are carrying a ball, with the left hand on top. Bring your right foot closer to the left foot, resting on the ball of the foot.

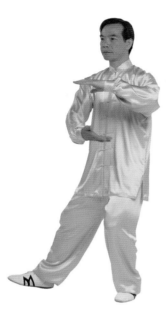

4 Step out to the right. Move the hands inwards slightly, as if squeezing the ball. This initiates the next movement.

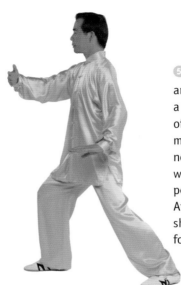

5 Push your right arm forward to form a semicircle in front of your chest and move your left hand next to your hip, with the fingers pointing forward. At the same time, shift your weight forward gradually.

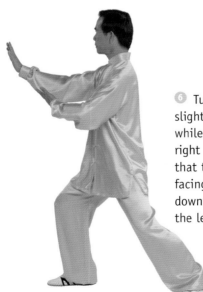

6 Turn your waist slightly to the right while turning your right hand out so that the palm is facing diagonally downwards. Turn the left palm up.

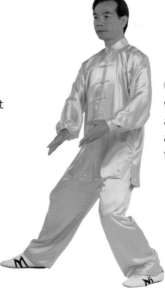

7 Shift your weight back and bring both arms down and to the left.

The 24 Forms
STROKING THE BIRD'S TAIL (RIGHT)

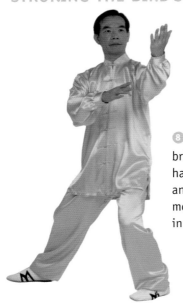

❽ Slowly bring both hands down and then up, moving them in gentle arcs.

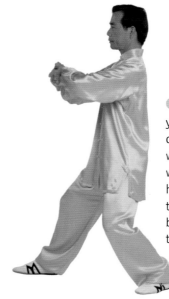

❾ Pressing your left palm onto your right wrist, shift your weight forward halfway and turn your body back to face the front.

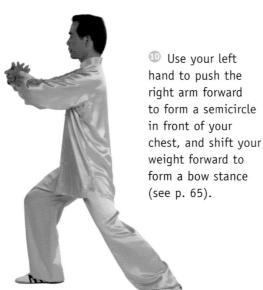

❿ Use your left hand to push the right arm forward to form a semicircle in front of your chest, and shift your weight forward to form a bow stance (see p. 65).

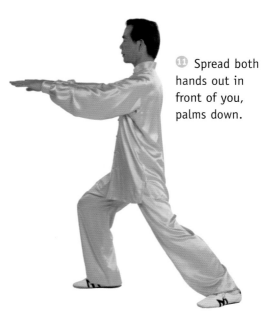

⓫ Spread both hands out in front of you, palms down.

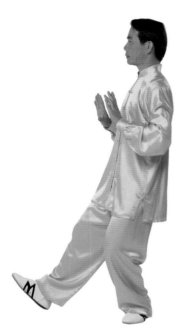

12 Bring your hands and weight back, and toes up, keeping your torso upright.

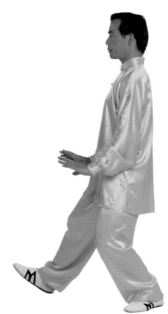

13 Bring your hands down in a gentle curve and sink the qi to the dan tian (or consciously think of the lower abdomen).

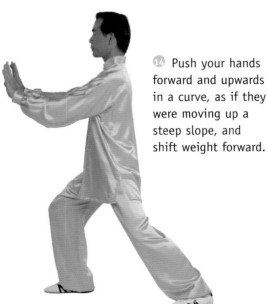

14 Push your hands forward and upwards in a curve, as if they were moving up a steep slope, and shift weight forward.

The 24 Forms

3 Movement 9
SINGLE WHIP

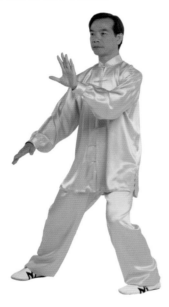

❶ Shift your weight back and turn your right toes inwards to face 12 o'clock. Move your right hand down, and move the left hand across slightly.

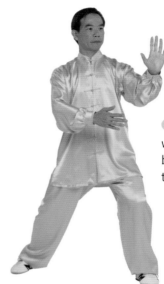

❷ Turning your waist, bring both hands to the left side.

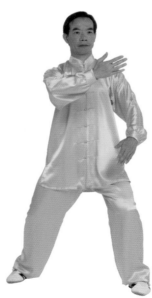

❸ Bring your right hand up and your left hand down.

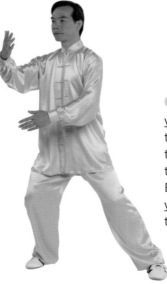

❹ Transferring your weight to the right, turn the waist to the right. Bring both your hands to the right.

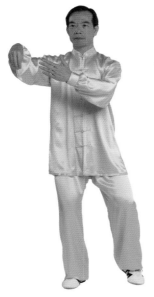

⑤ Turn the right palm out with the fingers pointing upwards, and then drop the fingers to make the right hand into a hook. Bring the left hand closer to the right, and the left foot closer to the right, resting on the ball of the foot.

HOOK HAND

Bring the fingers together with the fingertips pointing downwards. Bend the wrist to form a hook shape.

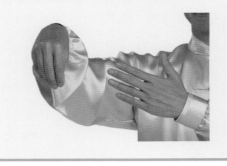

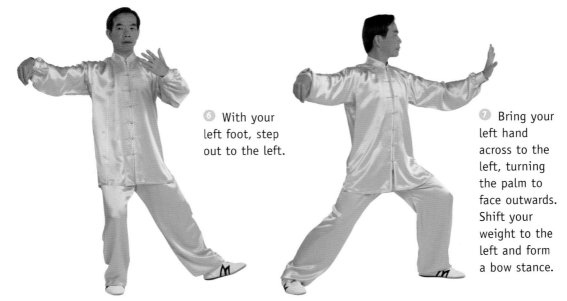

⑥ With your left foot, step out to the left.

⑦ Bring your left hand across to the left, turning the palm to face outwards. Shift your weight to the left and form a bow stance.

149

The 24 Forms

Movement 10
WAVING HANDS LIKE CLOUDS (THREE TIMES)

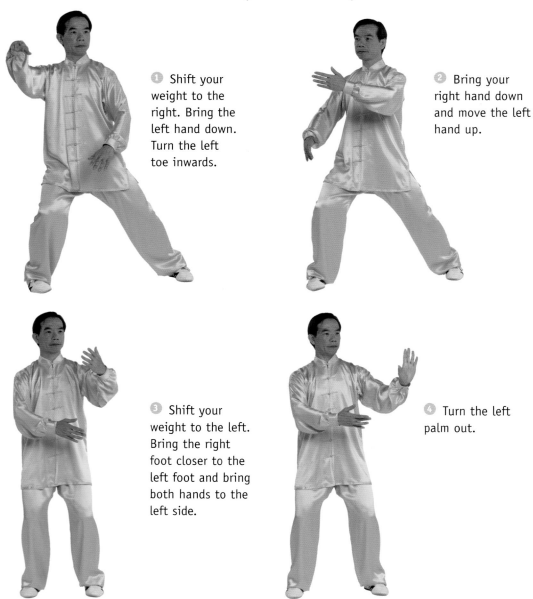

1 Shift your weight to the right. Bring the left hand down. Turn the left toe inwards.

2 Bring your right hand down and move the left hand up.

3 Shift your weight to the left. Bring the right foot closer to the left foot and bring both hands to the left side.

4 Turn the left palm out.

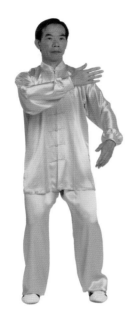

5 Bring your right hand up and move your left hand down. At the end, scoop up the left palm to face inwards.

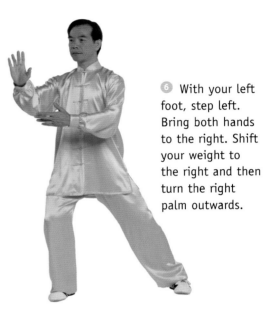

6 With your left foot, step left. Bring both hands to the right. Shift your weight to the right and then turn the right palm outwards.

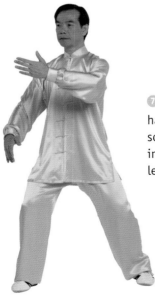

7 Bring your right hand down and scoop up to face inwards. Move your left hand up.

The 24 Forms

WAVING HANDS LIKE CLOUDS (THREE TIMES)

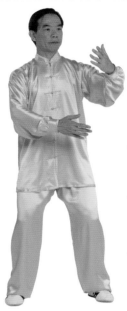

8 Shift your weight to the left. Bring your right foot closer to the left and move both hands to the left.

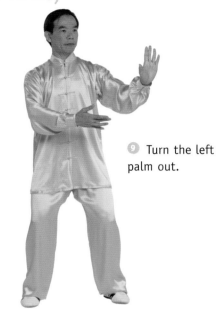

9 Turn the left palm out.

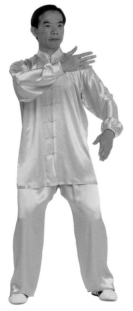

10 Bring the right palm up and left palm down.

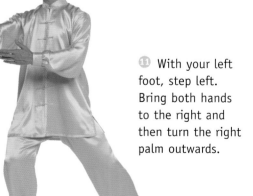

11 With your left foot, step left. Bring both hands to the right and then turn the right palm outwards.

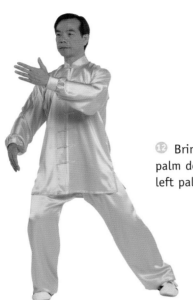

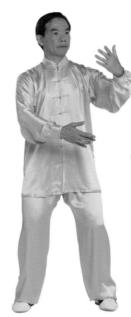

⑫ Bring the right palm down and the left palm up.

⑬ Shift your weight to the left. Bring the right foot closer to the left. Bring both hands to the left.

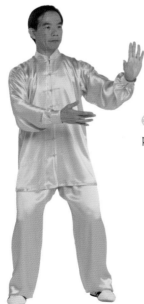

⑭ Turn the left palm out.

The 24 Forms

Movement 11
SINGLE WHIP

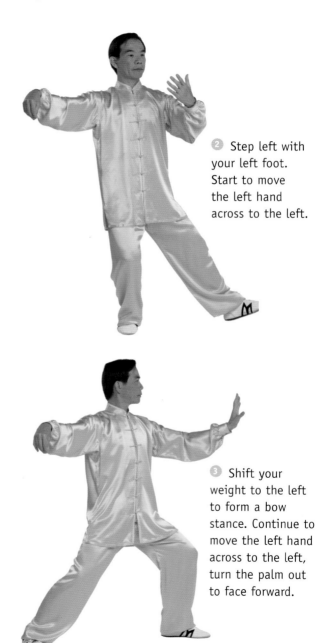

❷ Step left with
your left foot.
Start to move
the left hand
across to the left.

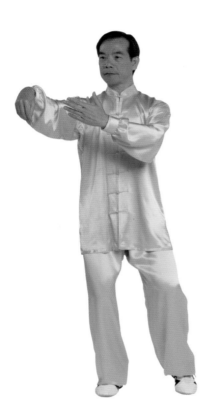

❸ Shift your
weight to the left
to form a bow
stance. Continue to
move the left hand
across to the left,
turn the palm out
to face forward.

❶ Bring both hands to the right.
Turn the right palm upwards and out
and then form a hook shape. Move the
left hand closer to the right, with the
palm facing inwards. Shift your weight
to the right and bring the left foot
closer to the right.

154

Movement 12
HIGH HORSE

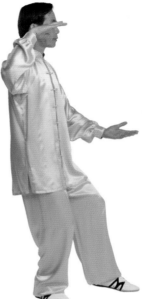

2 Bring the right hand close to the right ear. Bring the left palm back. Shift weight back to the right foot.

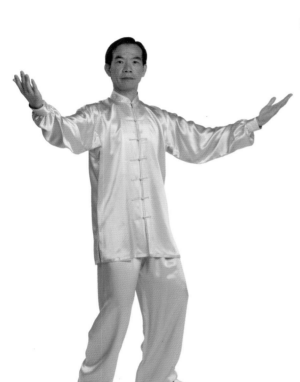

1 Open up both palms to face diagonally upwards and step half a step forward with the right foot.

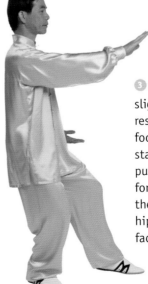

3 Shift the left foot slightly forward, then rest on the ball of the foot and form an empty stance. Continue to push the right hand forward and bring the left hand near your hip, with the palm facing upwards.

The 24 Forms

Movement 13
HEEL KICK (RIGHT)

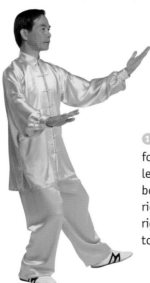

❶ With the left foot, step to the left. Open up both arms moving right hand to the right and left hand to the left.

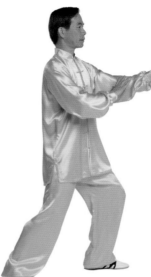

❷ Shift your weight onto the left. Move both hands in outward curves, bringing the right hand towards the left elbow.

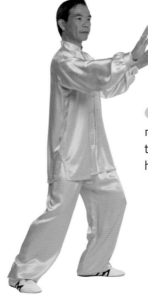

❸ Continue with the curves, moving the right hand across to the right and the left hand down towards the left.

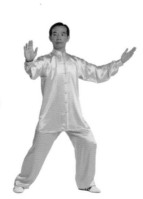

Front view

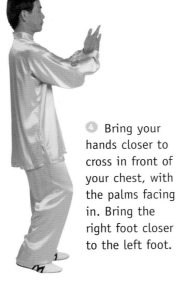

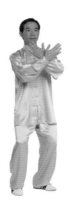

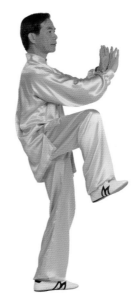

④ Bring your hands closer to cross in front of your chest, with the palms facing in. Bring the right foot closer to the left foot.

Front view

⑤ Turn both palms to face outwards, with the fingers pointing up. Bring the right knee up and lift up the toes of that foot.

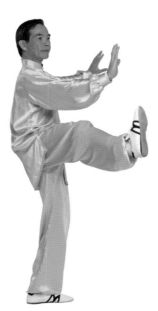

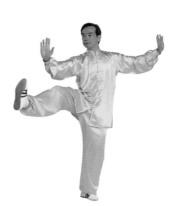

⑥ Kick out with the right heel while opening up both arms. Be sure to kick to a height that is comfortable for you. Keep your fingers pointing upwards and look at the right hand. Have your right hand pointing in the same direction as your right foot. Both palms are symmetrical, or the left hand could be slightly higher for better balance.

Front view

The 24 Forms

Movement 14
PUNCHING EARS WITH BOTH FISTS

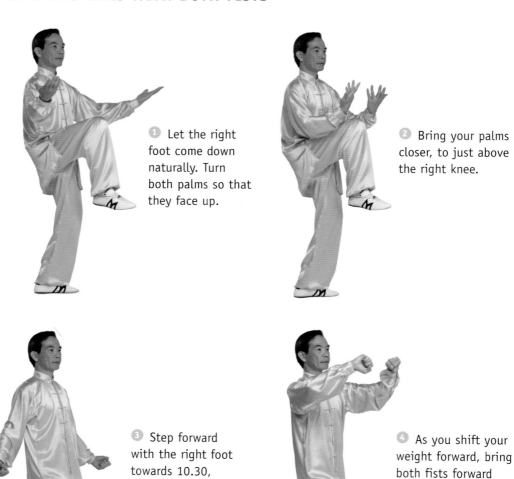

❶ Let the right foot come down naturally. Turn both palms so that they face up.

❷ Bring your palms closer, to just above the right knee.

❸ Step forward with the right foot towards 10.30, bringing both hands backwards to near your hip as you make them into fists.

❹ As you shift your weight forward, bring both fists forward as if punching someone's ears.

Movement 15
HEEL KICK (LEFT)

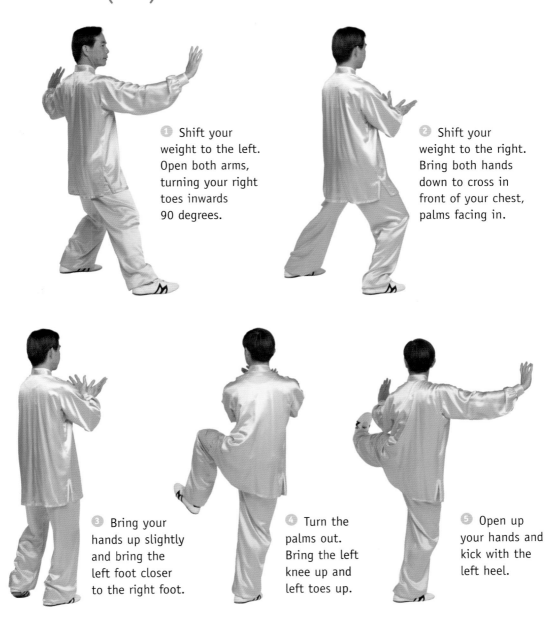

❶ Shift your weight to the left. Open both arms, turning your right toes inwards 90 degrees.

❷ Shift your weight to the right. Bring both hands down to cross in front of your chest, palms facing in.

❸ Bring your hands up slightly and bring the left foot closer to the right foot.

❹ Turn the palms out. Bring the left knee up and left toes up.

❺ Open up your hands and kick with the left heel.

The 24 Forms

Movement 16
LOWERING MOVEMENT AND GOLDEN COCK STANDING ON ONE LEG (LEFT)

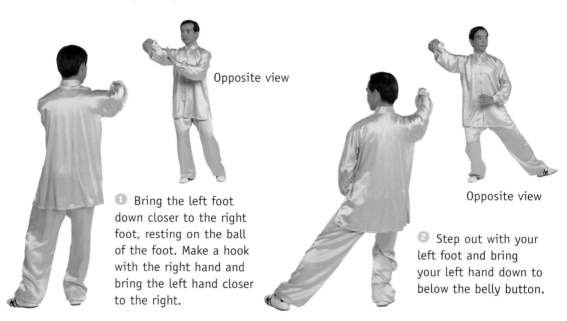

Opposite view

Opposite view

① Bring the left foot down closer to the right foot, resting on the ball of the foot. Make a hook with the right hand and bring the left hand closer to the right.

② Step out with your left foot and bring your left hand down to below the belly button.

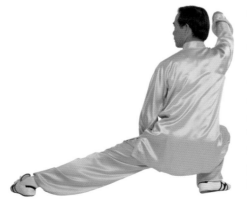

③ Lower your stance, keeping your weight on the right, then turn the left palm out. Make a hook with your right hand. This should all be done very carefully. Bend down only to your comfort level, while maintaining an upright posture. Keep both feet on the ground.

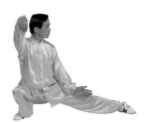

Opposite view

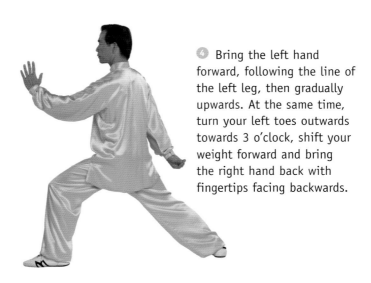

4 Bring the left hand forward, following the line of the left leg, then gradually upwards. At the same time, turn your left toes outwards towards 3 o'clock, shift your weight forward and bring the right hand back with fingertips facing backwards.

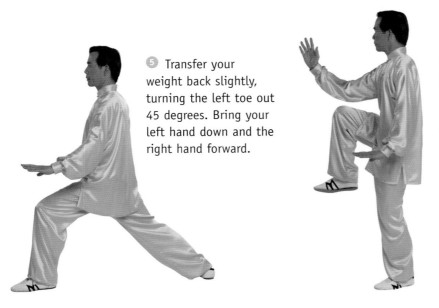

5 Transfer your weight back slightly, turning the left toe out 45 degrees. Bring your left hand down and the right hand forward.

6 Bring the right hand and right foot up. Move the left hand next to the hip.

161

The 24 Forms

Movement 17
LOWERING MOVEMENT AND GOLDEN COCK STANDING ON ONE LEG (RIGHT)

1 Gently touch down with the right foot, turning the toes slightly inwards (in a pigeon-toed fashion). Make a left-hand hook and bring the right hand across.

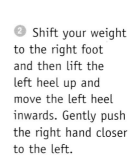

2 Shift your weight to the right foot and then lift the left heel up and move the left heel inwards. Gently push the right hand closer to the left.

3 Step out with the right foot and bring the right hand down.

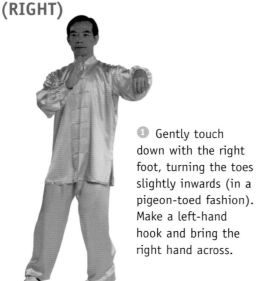

4 Lower your stance to your comfort level and turn the right palm out.

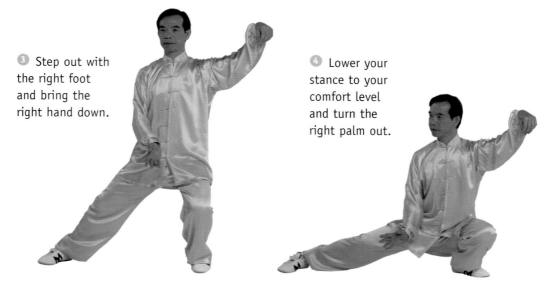

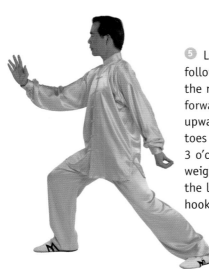

⑤ Let your right hand follow the line of the right leg, moving forward and then upwards. Turn your toes outwards towards 3 o'clock. Shift your weight forward while the left hand forms a hook hand.

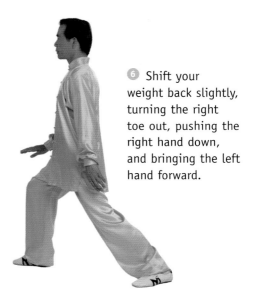

⑥ Shift your weight back slightly, turning the right toe out, pushing the right hand down, and bringing the left hand forward.

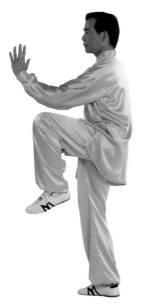

⑦ Lift the left hand up to eye level and lift the left knee up.

The 24 Forms

7 ★ Movement 18
FAIR LADY WORKING AT THE SHUTTLES (RIGHT AND LEFT)

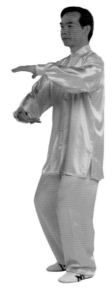

❶ Bring the left foot down at an angle of 45 degrees (1.30 position). Put the weight on the left foot and bring the right foot closer to the left. Place your hands as if you were carrying a ball, with the left hand on top.

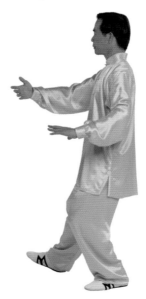

❷ With the right foot, step towards your right side (toes pointing at 4.30). Separate the hands.

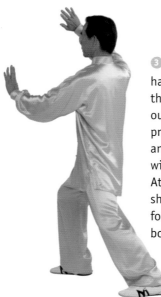

❸ Bring the right hand around, with the palm facing outwards, to protect your head, and push forward with the left hand. At the same time, shift your weight forward to form a bow stance.

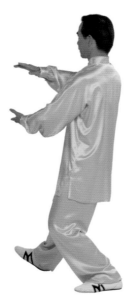

❹ Shift your weight backwards. Lift the right toe up and then down in the same spot. Position your hands as if they were carrying a ball with right hand on top.

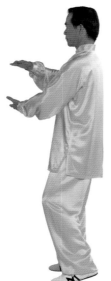

5 With your weight on the right foot, bring the left foot closer to the right.

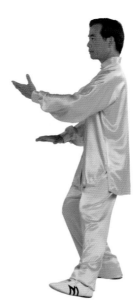

6 Step to the left, pointing your foot towards 1.30. Separate your hands.

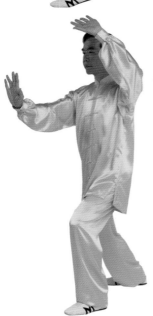

7 Bring the left hand around, palm outwards, to protect your head, and push forward with the right hand.

The 24 Forms

Movement 19
NEEDLE AT THE BOTTOM SEA

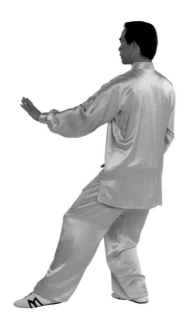 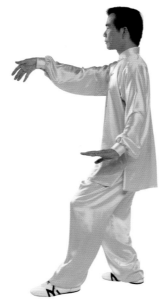 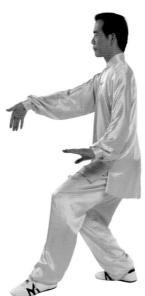

❶ Take half a step forward with the right foot. Turn very slightly to the right. Bring both hands towards the right.

❷ When the left hand reaches the midline, slowly press down. At the same time, lift up the right hand with the fingers pointing down, then turn slightly back to face the left and move your left hand near your hip. At the same time, move right hand forward. Move the left foot forward slightly to make an empty stance.

❸ Lower your stance (by bending the right knee and hip) to within your comfort level, pushing the right hand down.

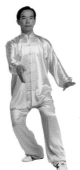

Front view

Movement 20
FAN (BACK)

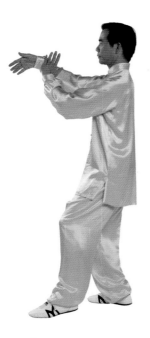 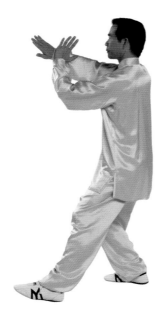 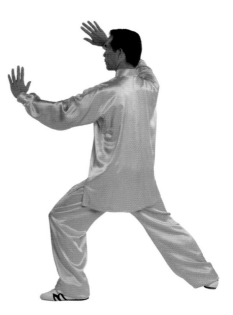

❶ Lift up your right hand. Bring your left hand up so that the left hand is pressing on the right wrist, and stand up.

❷ Take half a step forward with the left foot. Turn the right palm out.

❸ Open up both hands like a fan and shift your weight forward to form a bow stance.

The 24 Forms

Movement 21
TURN TO DEFLECT DOWNWARDS, PARRY AND PUNCH

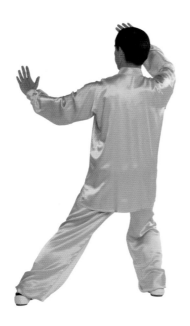 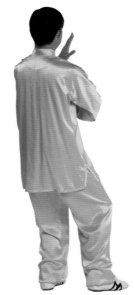 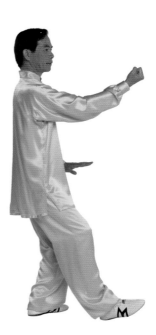

❶ Turn towards the right. Turn the left toes in as much as you can. Bring both hands to the right.

❷ Move your left hand on top, and place the right hand just in front of the left armpit. Shift weight onto left foot. Bring the right foot closer to the left.

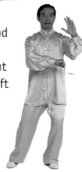

Opposite view

❸ Bring the right fist upwards and the left hand down to the hip. Step the right foot down with toes turning inwards.

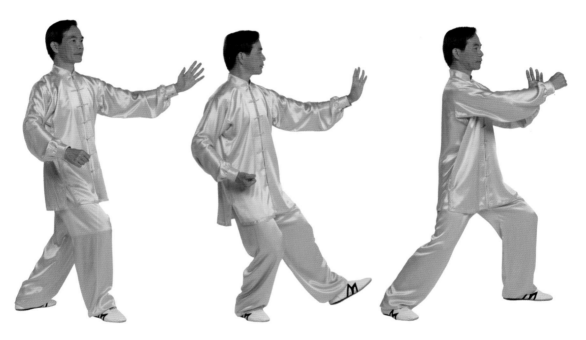

④ Shift your weight forward. Bring your right hand to near the hip and "scoop up" with the left hand as if you're going to embrace somebody.

⑤ Step forward with the left foot. Rotate your right fist so that the palm faces forward.

⑥ Move your weight forward. Punch forward and at the same time rotate the right fist slowly, ending with the thumb facing upwards. Bring the left hand over and move it along the right wrist.

The 24 Forms

Movement 22
APPARENT CLOSING UP

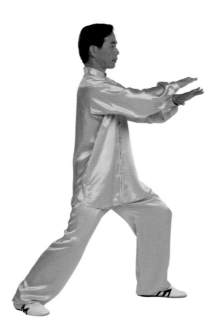

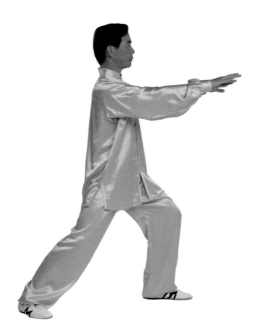

❶ Open up your right fist and move the left hand under the right elbow, then move it forward.

❷ Separate your hands to shoulder width.

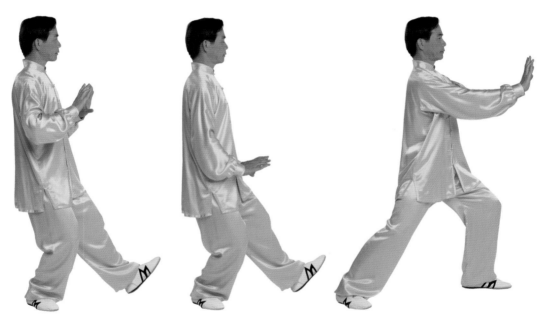

③ Bring your weight back and your hands back, turning the palms to face forward.

④ Push your hands down gently.

⑤ Push your hands forward and upwards and move your weight forward.

The 24 Forms

Movement 23
CROSS HANDS

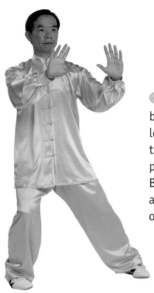

① Shift your weight backwards. Turn the left toe inwards so that the toes are pointing forward. Bring your hands across in front of you.

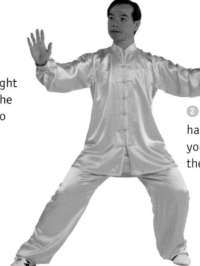

② Separate your hands. Transfer your weight to the left.

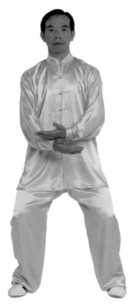

③ Bring your hands down and cross them, with the palms facing up. Bring the right foot closer so that both feet are shoulder-width apart and both sets of toes are pointing forward.

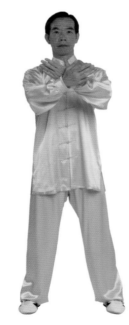

④ Slowly stand up. Bring your hands up in front of your chest.

Movement 24
CLOSING FORM

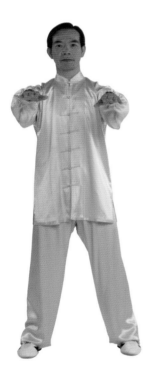 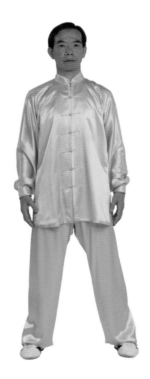 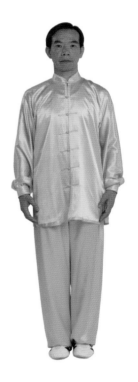

❶ Separate your hands.

❷ Bring your hands down slowly to rest beside your legs.

❸ Bring your feet together.

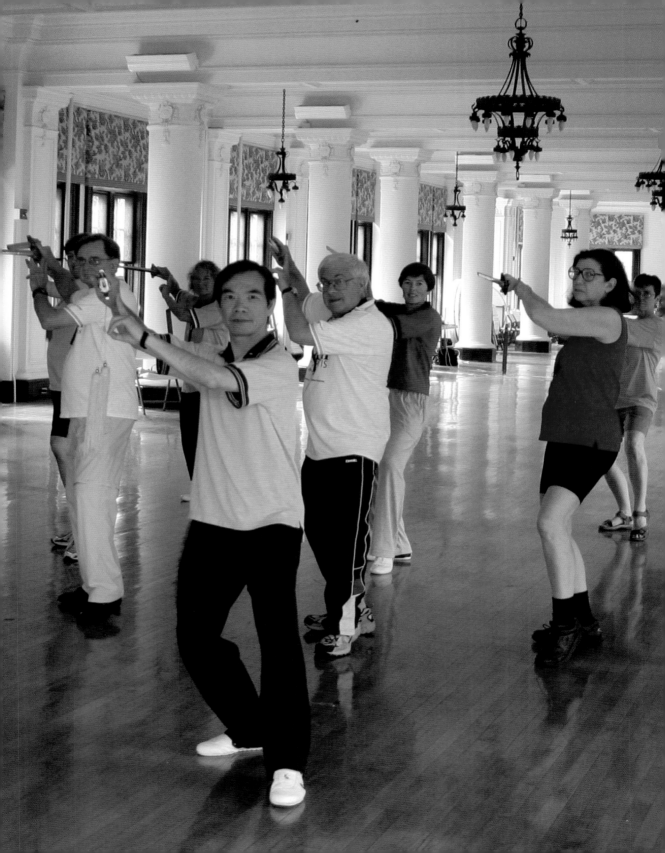

PART 3

BEYOND THE 24 FORMS

CHAPTER 8

HOW TO IMPROVE YOUR TAI CHI

After learning the Tai Chi Beginner's Set and the 24 Forms, you will have a good foundation in tai chi and will have reached what we might call an intermediate level. Going beyond this will take you to a high level, which will bring you even more pleasure and even greater health benefits.

How you proceed depends on your interests and personality. People learn differently. You might prefer to concentrate on the forms you have already learned, or instead branch out and learn new sets. Either approach can take you to a higher level, as long as you continue to practise regularly.

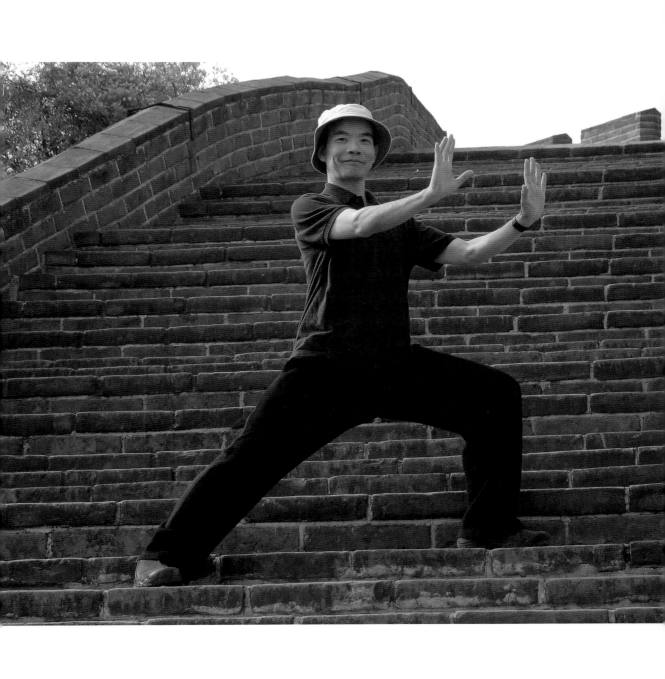

Tai chi is not a sport in which progress is measured by a standardized grading system or points or wins accumulated in competition. Instead progress is marked by an increasing sense of personal fulfilment, ever-greater enjoyment of practice, a feeling of wellness and strength, and markedly better health.

What do people mean when they refer to "a high level of tai chi"? Is it a matter of how many sets of forms you learn? Is it a particular martial-art ability? Or is it the colour of a medal won in competition? The answer depends on your values. It's partly a matter of what you want to get out of tai chi. But for us, the most important measurement is how well you understand the essential tai chi principles and how well you've integrated them into your practice.

Take Val, for example. She started tai chi when she was so riddled with arthritis she could barely stand. She used a wheelchair and could only walk about five or six metres without it. But after only six months of tai chi, she was able to get rid of her wheelchair. Although every now and then she still had pain, she was enjoying the same mobility and lifestyle as most of her friends of the same age. Since then she has kept up with her tai chi practice on a regular basis. She continues to improve, without needing the challenge of "higher forms". She has incorporated the essential principles into her practice to the best of her physical ability. Her tai chi forms contain depth and have a good balance of internal and external components. More important, she enjoys her tai chi, which has helped her to be much more mobile, healthier and more serene. It has even given her the confidence to start teaching others, to help them improve their health, too.

In our opinion, Val has reached a high level of tai chi. Indeed, we are sure she has in her own way achieved more than many younger, stronger, more flexible practitioners, even some who have learned many sets of forms. Being able to perform low stances and raise your leg to a great height may look impressive, but it stands for little if it isn't accompanied by the substantial internal developments that should also be derived from the practice of tai chi, such as looseness and serenity.

In high-level tai chi, albeit to varying degrees, tai chi becomes a way of life for the practitioner. Sun Lu-tang, the creator of the Sun style and one of the greatest martial artists in history, said that the highest level of tai chi is not being invincible, but is achieving the Dao. The Dao is nature. In other words, the practitioner reaches the highest level of tai chi when he or she is in harmony within himself or herself and with nature. At a high level of tai chi, it is this internal component that matters most.

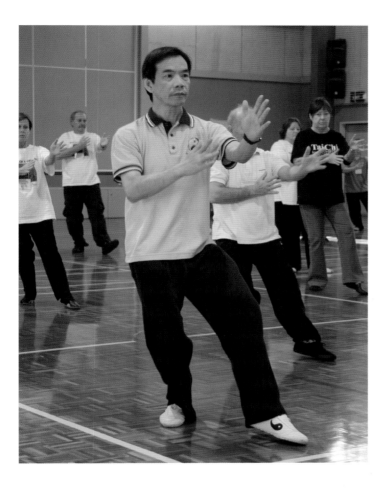

It's not necessary to learn any more sets of tai chai than the 24 Forms in order to reach a high level. We had one tai chi teacher tell us: "Over the last 30 years, I've learned many sets of forms. My greatest improvement came from teaching the simple sets of forms like the Tai Chi Beginner's Set. When I teach how to integrate the essential principles into these simple sets, I demonstrate. And as I demonstrate, I focus on integrating the principles. Through the numerous repetitions, I found that my understanding of the essential principles deepened each time, and as a result, my forms improved immensely."

So, as you can see, you can become a high-level tai chi practitioner using just the 24 Forms.

Learning new sets

However, the saying "curiosity killed the cat" doesn't hold true for tai chi. There's no harm in learning other styles. Indeed, exposures to other forms or styles might just help you reach a higher level. For many people, obtaining different perspectives on an activity can provide a better understanding of the whole.

Often, tai chi beginners ask, "Is there only one absolute right way?" We don't think so. Given that there are so many great tai chi practitioners who use different styles and

forms, it's likely that there are many right ways. Many roads lead to Rome.

Consider the differences between classic styles. In Yang style, you move forward and backwards by lifting your foot just off the ground and touching down like a "cat". In Chen style, you step forward, brushing your foot on the ground and often stomping noisily on the ground. If you have learned Yang style, you might think Chen stylists are all wrong!

"Depress the chest and raise the upper back" is one of the 10 essential points made by Yang Chen-fu (which are widely regarded as some of the most important tai chi principles). But what does that mean? Some Yang stylists take this to mean that they should hunch their backs; others don't, believing it means you should relax the chest and let the internal force reach the back.

Different styles even have different hand shapes. For example, Yang style uses an open palm, while Chen uses a more closed one. Even within one style, you might encounter many variations and even significant differences.

All of this tells us that these minor differences, although they might add to the challenge or enjoyment of tai chi, aren't important. The crucial thing is to understand and integrate the essential principles of tai chi, which are similar in all styles.

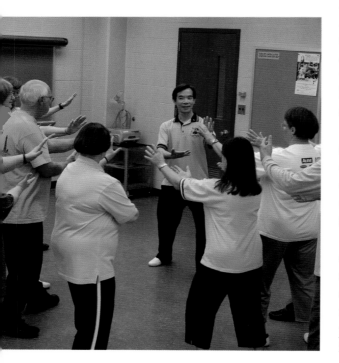

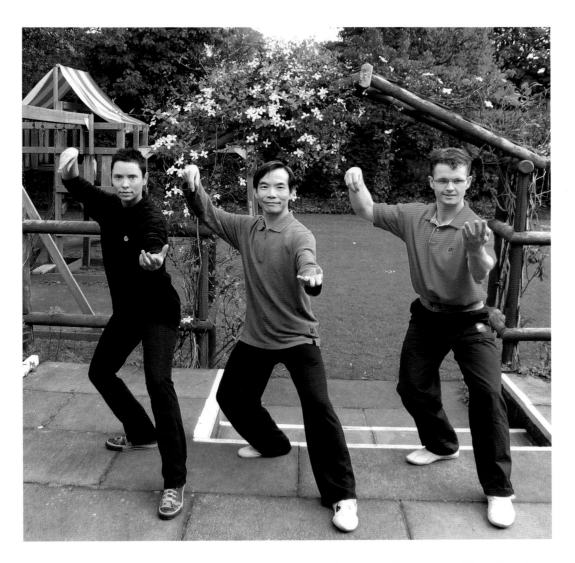

It's challenging and fun to continue to strive for a higher level in tai chi, but it's important to understand that no-one knows everything about tai chi and that no-one is perfect. The enjoyment and benefits come from the journey of progression. Only through regular practice will you truly understand the inner meaning of tai chi, and make the most of its potential benefits. So make that your top priority.

Whichever route you decide to take towards high-level tai chi, the following information will guide you along the way.

Extending the essential principles

To really improve your tai chi, look at incorporating four other essential concepts: *jing*, *song*, *chen*, and *huo*. These are an extension of the essential tai chi principles discussed in Chapter 4 (see p. 112). The following repeats some of that information but explores it in different and deeper ways.

The four concepts complement each other, so you don't need to be completely proficient in one before moving on to another. They also affect each other positively, so that by learning more about one you will improve your understanding of the others. Try working on one concept for a period of at least a few weeks and then move on to another. But come back to each one regularly.

Some of the concepts might not be clear to you initially. Don't let that concern you. As you progress further, you'll be able to understand them. In time, as your level of understanding deepens, the words will take on a somewhat different meaning. Bear in mind that no-one reaches perfection in all four concepts; here, too, progression is what matters.

Jing

Jing, roughly translated, means "mental quietness". To attain this quietness of the mind, imagine yourself in a tranquil environment such as a shady rainforest. Your mind is serene but you are still aware of the surroundings.

As you practise tai chi, try to put yourself in that mental state. A good way to facilitate this is to focus on one movement at a time. Try to focus on one essential principle (see p. 112) at a time. Practise it, together with mental quietness from within, for a length of time, and then move onto the next principle.

Attaining a degree of mental quietness will take time. But once you have achieved it, your mind will retain a memory of that state. The next time you practise, your mind will be able to recall that same state relatively quickly, so that you won't have to start from scratch again. And, as you practise more, you'll be able to move on to a higher level each time.

A good way to help yourself return to the same mental state is to use a key word. Whenever you are practising to attain jing, say the word "jing" over and over in your head. Then, when you start the next practice session, repeating the word to yourself will help to return you to the same state.

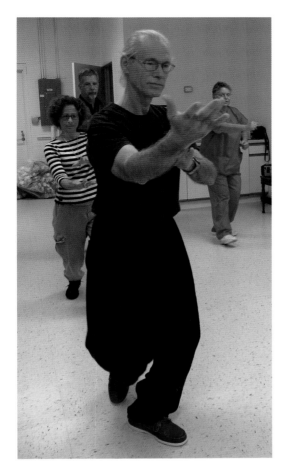

Jing improves relaxation and enhances concentration. This, in turn, relieves muscle tension and improves your coordination, making your tai chi practice more effective.

The mental quietness of tai chi is different from that of some forms of meditation where people are placed in a secluded environment. While you're serene from within, you're still aware of your environment and able to assess the situation around you at any time—which is essential when you're performing tai chi as a martial art. It's like having a small world within yourself and yet you are still very much in the bigger real world around you. Using Jing state will help you deal with not only a martial-art fight but with various crises in real life.

Song

Song is often translated as "relaxation", but it means more than that in Chinese, conveying a sense of loosening and stretching out. Imagine all your joints loosening, stretching out or expanding gently from within. Take your shoulder joint, for example. If you gently stretch out that joint, you'll feel a small dimple on the top of the shoulder. If you tense the shoulder joint, the dimple disappears.

You can apply this technique to other joints, too. Visualize them loosening. In the upper limbs, loosen your elbows, wrists and finger joints by stretching them out from within. In the torso, the loosening should be vertical—visualize your spine as a string that you gently stretch from both ends. For the lower limbs, stretch your hip joints and knee joints gently outwards, so that your crouch forms an arch shape.

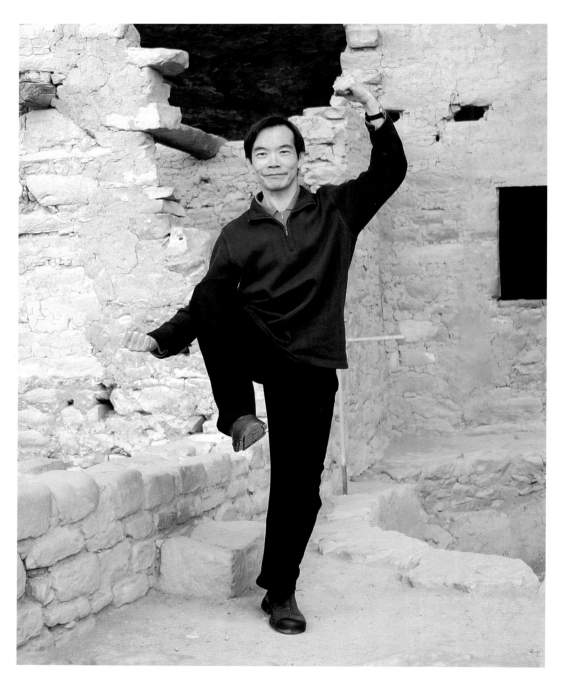

This method of loosening constitutes a type of controlled relaxation, because when you gently stretch your joints, you release tension. "Song" helps your qi flow, builds internal strength and also improves flexibility. It will also enhance "jing". The more your body develops song, the more your mind becomes jing, and as your mind becomes more jing, it further enhances your song, thus setting up a positive circle.

Chen

Chen (not the same word in Chinese as the name of the Chen-style) means "sinking". As you progress in tai chi, you'll come across the term "sinking your qi to the dan tian". An area three fingerwidths below the belly button, the dan tian is central to everything we do in tai chi (see p. 99).

Exhaling facilitates the sinking of qi to the dan tian, which in turn keeps your mind jing and loosens up your joints. You'll find using the abdominal breathing method (see p. 55) will help you to feel the sensation of qi. As you breathe out, loosen your joints. You should feel a warm, heavy feeling in your dan tian. That's the feeling of sinking your qi. If you don't feel this initially, don't worry. Continue to practise the form as best you can, and coordinate your breathing with the movement. Be aware of your dan tian area during the exhalation. As you improve

your tai chi, you'll eventually feel the qi in the dan tian and learn how to sink it.

To chen well, one needs to be song and jing. The right mental state, combined with the loosening of the joints and an out breath, is the most effective way to achieve chen.

Chen enhances stability, song and qi cultivation. Awareness of the dan tian will also strengthen the internal structures of your body and improve your inner strength.

Huo

Huo means "agility", being able to move nimbly. Being strong, having powerful qi, and being in a good mental state are essential for good tai chi, and these attributes will be even more effective when you also have good huo.

Agility comes mainly from regular practice, utilizing the proper body posture and weight transference, good control of movements, loosened joints, and strong internal strength. Agility also aids qi cultivation and improves flexibility.

Strategies for self-improvement

We've made it clear that to improve your tai chi you must understand the tai chi principles and practise regularly and with awareness. Now let's look at some other methods that will help you improve your skills. Some of these will work more effectively for some learners than for others, but they should help most people.

Getting beyond the plateau phase

In his book *Mastery: The Keys to Success and Long-Term Fulfillment*, George Leonard, a well-known California martial-art expert, describes the concept of the "plateau phase". He explains that learners go through phases. In between each quantum leap of technical advancement, there's a long period during which improvement is slow and not obvious. This is the plateau phase, which is necessary for absorbing knowledge and skill before the next phase of rapid advancement can happen.

A typical learning curve for tai chi therefore looks like this:

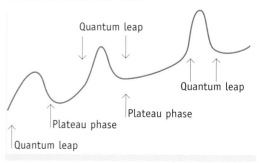

Quantum leap

Quantum leap

Plateau phase

Plateau phase

Quantum leap

Steep rises are separated by wide plateaus. Impatient students become bored and disappointed during the plateau phases and often drop out.

In tai chi, plateaus and steep rises are yin and yang. The former involves storing energy and the latter involves delivering energy—you need to store energy before you can deliver it. In the long run, being aware of and learning how to enjoy the plateaus will help you persist and make progress. Learning about the concept of flow can help you enjoy the plateau phase more.

Getting your flow going

Flow occurs when a person is so absorbed or so fully engaged in an activity that he or she becomes "lost in time". It often happens when an athlete performs at his or her best, or when an artist paints a masterpiece. Athletes sometimes call it "being in the zone". Whether you are doing a job, hobby or sport—or tai chi—if you are fully engaged, you are more likely to be "in flow".

After years of studying many thousands of people, Professor Mihaly Csikszentmihalyi, a professor of psychology at the University of Chicago and the author of *Finding Flow: The Psychology of Engagement with Everyday Life*, has found a close connection between enjoyment and flow. People whose lives are fulfilled and serene are more often in flow.

He also found that it is possible to increase flow, and these findings are well supported by other experts.

Knowing that more flow leads to more enjoyment and fulfilment in life, you can work to increase your flow. If you can enjoy what you're doing, you know you will do better. Being more often in flow also means your tai chi will be better.

Three main factors can induce flow:

1 having a clear goal or goals
2 receiving immediate and relevant feedback
3 matching your goals to your skills

A "goal" in this case means a short-term goal. For example, your goal for one round of practice could be to move smoothly, or simply to remember the movement. You'll know right away if you have remembered your movements correctly and if they're smooth. In other words, you will get immediate and relevant feedback.

By carefully matching your goals to your skill level, you can increase your chances of achieving flow. If you're a newcomer to tai chi and unfamiliar with the moves, trying to do them smoothly could be too difficult and that may cause stress, which could in turn stop you from entering the flow state. On the other hand, if you're experienced in tai chi, you may already be doing your moves smoothly, so this goal may offer no challenge at all, and that could also prevent you from entering the flow state. To facilitate flow, you need to set a goal that is sufficiently challenging but not likely to cause frustration.

In tai chi, we aim to integrate body and mind, which can take you to a mental state similar to flow. As your tai chi improves, you'll be in flow more often. More flow will bring you more enjoyment, more enjoyment will drive you to practise more, and more practice will result in more flow.

Feeling good naturally

The human body resonates with nature and tai chi follows the rhythms of nature, so it should make you feel in tune with nature and feel good. Try to work natural flows and rhythms into your practice.

Learning new skills

Learning something new often stimulates people to try harder. We've observed that among students who come from all over the world to our annual one-week tai chi workshops. At the end of the workshops, they demonstrate what they've learned. The sparkle in their eyes from these demonstrations indicates their pride and pleasure. Whether you're learning a new set of forms or improving your forms, you're learning a new skill. Recognize and feel the excitement of that.

Helping people

Many tai chi practitioners around the world teach tai chi. Why? Most do it for the enjoyment they get out of helping people improve their health and quality of life. Helping others is a powerful motivator, so try to teach whenever you can. Teaching is also one of the best ways to improve your own skills.

Getting the habit

As humans are creatures of habit, it's easy to make a routine of regular practice—the key to improving tai chi. Set a time for daily practice. Once you get into the habit, you'll find that your mind and body will demand it.

Feeling better

Many scientific studies have shown the health benefits of tai chi. Numerous people have made significant improvements in their health and quality of life by practising it. And the point is, they've done it themselves. They've taken control of improving their own life situations. In turn, the health benefits and the pride people feel as a result drive them to further improve their tai chi.

Using mind power

Tai chi is an internal art, which means that you have to use your thinking ability. And this is a big part of what makes tai chi so interesting. Use your thinking power in your practice. Analyze your moves. What is the intrinsic purpose of the move? Does it make good sense? Does it feel comfortable? Does it feel balanced? Is it consistent with tai chi principles? Does it give you a stronger feeling of qi? Is it safe? Be aware of your body and focus your mind. Analyzing your own tai chi is the best way to gain deeper understanding and make improvements.

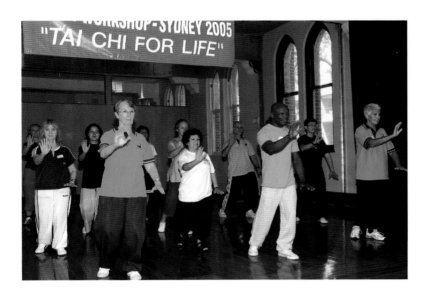

Using your mind also means allowing your mind to be open. If you're fixed on one idea and have closed your mind to others, then your mind is like a full cup: it can't take in anything else. It's closed. Only when it's open or empty, can it can take in more material, and only then will you progress.

Absorbing

You must digest your food to make it useful to your body. You also have to digest tai chi until it gets inside your body, into your bones, and becomes a part of you. When you learn new techniques or forms, you should try to practise them until you have fully digested them. Only after digestion can you expand the skill.

Using self-guided imagery

One recently developed technique that has proved highly useful for learning disciplines such as tai chi is self-guided imagery. This is a way of training your unconscious mind which has been used by many athletes to improve their performance. With some modifications, it can be used to improve tai chi skills and to help you remember the forms. For a full explanation, consult the article on this topic by Dr Paul Lam and Dr Yanchy Lacska in the Appendix, p. 196.

Letting go

This idea was summed up nicely in an inspiring talk by Sheila Rae, a tai chi and qigong teacher: "There comes a point in our practice where we must learn to let go of the form, the perfectionism, and of the ego." Letting go and allowing nature to take effect can be a very useful approach at particular times. For more information, see the full text of Sheila's talk in the Appendix, p. 202.

Working with a teacher

Sooner or later, if you're to progress to a higher level, you'll realize that you'll need a teacher. Face-to-face instruction from a suitable teacher can enhance your tai chi immeasurably. On the other hand, an unsuitable teacher can set you back. People we know have given up tai chi because they've had unsuitable teachers. So take your time to find a teacher with whom you click and who will meet your needs.

A good teacher can guide you to reach your goal in tai chi no matter what stage you're at. If your new teacher starts by saying, "Everything you've learned thus far is all wrong, you've wasted your time", consider looking for another teacher.

If you live in a fairly large community, chances are you won't have much trouble locating a few teachers. Ask your friends for recommendations. (You can also consult Dr Lam's website at www.taichiproductions.com, which includes a list of instructors worldwide.) Make contact with the teachers. Find out what style of tai chi each one teaches. Does he or she take beginners or other levels? What's the charge? Ask if you can observe the teacher leading a class. That can give you vital information that will help you make your decision.

When you visit a class, watch the students, and if possible talk to them. Do they seem interested and enthusiastic? Do they ask the teacher questions and get a satisfactory response? Are their objectives similar to yours? Are there regular students?

Margaret Brade, LlB, BSc, MBA, CEO of Age Concern Stockport, UK, and a tai chi teacher, says this of her own teacher: "[Bruce] had some magic for me—and many others. It is hard to capture in words what someone has that makes 30-plus people turn up twice a week, week after week—all those instructors that have come after him (he has now retired) have not managed it, and people still constantly talk of Bruce."

Take a look at the list of precautions in Chapter 2 (pp. 25–6). Does the teacher show concern for issues such as these? Are warm-up and cooling-down exercises part of the program? Is the teacher more interested in martial art or health?

Finding a teacher might be more difficult if you live in a small town. You might have to resort to taking workshops or using instructional DVDs or videos and books rather than attending ongoing classes. However, in addition to regular home-based classes, many excellent tai chi teachers travel around the world giving courses. You can often find out about these courses, or workshops, online.

In the tai chi world, it's not uncommon to come across teachers who teach in what's called a "traditional manner"—in other words, they're from the "old school". Many such teachers expect their students to learn simply by following them; they don't provide instruction. They may even discourage two-way communication or be negative about a student's progress. Some traditional teachers also demand total loyalty; in other words, you're not allowed to obtain instruction from another person or even from materials such as books and DVDs. Nowadays, however, these teachers are becoming rare.

This isn't to say that the traditional-style teacher is all bad. Many traditionally oriented teachers have much to offer. Whether you opt for this kind of instruction depends on your understanding, tolerance, how you learn best, and whether you have any choice.

MAKING THE MOST OF CLASSES

Once you decide to study with a teacher, you can get more out of your classes by keeping the following suggestions in mind.

■ Always try to understand your teacher, and his or her objectives and methodology. Open your mind and be receptive. Show respect, which will help you connect with your teacher.

■ Be prepared for corrections, negative feedback and even criticism. Remember that many teachers are particularly hard on talented students because they expect more from them. If you see it in that light when your teacher is critical of you, you can treat it as positive feedback!

■ Prepare for your lessons so that you get more out of them. Find out what the next lesson holds in store and get ready for it. That way you'll absorb more information on the day.

There may come a time when you feel you've learned as much as you can from your teacher. It may then be time for you to make a change. Don't feel guilty. Each teacher has something different to offer. Why not take advantage of that fact? Simply let the teacher know in a respectful way, show your appreciation, and be honest about why you are leaving.

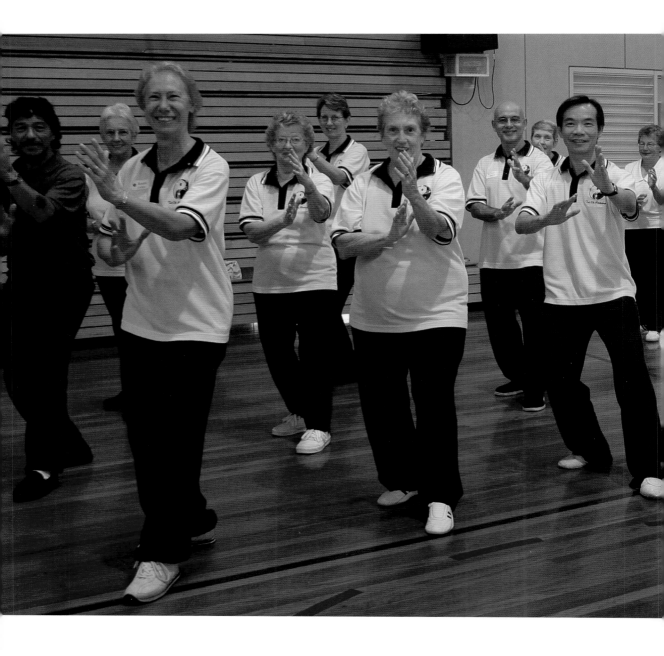

PART 4

RESOURCES

References

Books

These books are listed in order of preference by the author.

Overcoming Arthritis, Dr Paul Lam and Judith Horstman, Dorling Kindersley, Melbourne, 2002.

Simplified Taijiquan, China Sports Series 1, compiled by the China Sports Editorial Board, Beijing, China, 1990.

Xing Yi Quan Xue, The Study of Form—Mind Boxing, Sun Lu Tang, translated by Albert Liu, compiled and edited by Dan Miller, High View Publication, 1993.

The Essence of T'ai Chi Ch'uan—The Literary Tradition, translated and edited by Benjamin Pang Jeng Lo, Martin Inn, Robert Amacker and Susan Foe, North Atlantic Books, Berkeley, California, 1979.

The Taijiquan Classics, Barbara Davis, North Atlantic Books, Berkeley, California, USA.

Nei Jia Quan: Internal Martial Art, edited by Jess O'Brien, North Atlantic Books, 2004. (Interviews with masters on the internal component.)

Tai Chi as a Path of Wisdom, Linda Myoki Lehrhaupt, Shambala Publications, Boston and London, 2001.

The Complete Idiot's Guide to Tai Chi and Qigong, Bill Douglas, Alpha Books, 1633 Broadway, New York, NY, 2002.

Ride the Tiger to the Mountain—Tai Chi for Health, Martin and Emily Lee and JoAn Johnstone, Perseus Books Reading, Massachusetts, 1989.

The Inner Structure of Tai Chi, Mantak Chia and Juan Li, Healing Tao Books, Huntington, NY, 1996

Yang Style Taijiquan, compiled by Morning Glory Press, Hai Feng Publishing Co. Hong Kong, 1988.

Chen Style Taijiquan, compiled by Zhaohua Publishing House, Hong Kong, Hai Feng Publishing Co., Hong Kong, 1984.

Taiji: 48 Forms and Swordplay, China Sports Series 3, compiled by China Sports Editorial Board, Beijing, China, 1988.

Cheng Man-Ch'ing's Advanced T'ai-Chi Form Instruction, compiled and translated by Douglas Wile, Sweet Chi Press, Brooklyn, NY, 1985.

Destructive Emotions, How We Can Overcome Them, the Dalai Lama and Daniel Goleman, Bantam Books.

Arts of Strength, Arts of Serenity, Nicklaus Suino, Weatherhill Inc., New York, NY, 1996.

The Complete System of Self Healing: Internal Exercises, Dr Stephen T. Chang, Tao Publishing.

Taoist Meditation, The Mao-Shan (Shang-ch'ing) Tradition of Great Purity, Isabelle Robinet, State University of New York Press.

Tai Chi Ch'uan—The Technique of Power, Tem Horwitz and Susan Kimmelman, Rider and Company, London, 1979.

Magazines

T'ai Chi—The International Magazine of T'ai Chi Chuan
Wayfarer Publications
PO Box 39938
Los Angeles, CA 90039-0938, USA

Qi—The Journal of Traditional Eastern Health and Fitness
Insight Publishing Inc.
PO Box 18476
Anaheim Hills, CA 9281, USA

Organizations

Tai Chi Association of Australia—working together to promote tai chi in Australia www.taichiaustralia.com

Tai Chi for Health Community— based in USA, a non-profit organization dedicated to bringing tai chi to people in the interests of health improvement. www.taichiforhealthcommunity.org.

Better Health Tai Chi Chuan, Inc.— based in Australia, a non-profit organization aiming to share tai chi with as many people as possible. www.betterhealthtcc.com.au

World Tai Chi & Qigong Day—the biggest event in tai chi worldwide, organized by Bill Douglas: www.worldtaichiday.org

Tai Chi America—provides a multimedia learning resource and archive for all interested in tai chi chuan and chi kung: www.taichiamerica.com/

Tai Chi Union in UK—the UK tai chi association: www.taichiunion.com/

DVDs, videos and websites

Dr Paul Lam's teams of experts has produced several series of tai chi DVDs and videos from introductory teach-yourself series for health, to the advanced series to expand your skill. Below are the most popular titles:

Tai Chi for Beginners (available in English, Chinese, French, Spanish, German and Italian)

Tai Chi for Arthritis (available in English, Chinese, French, Spanish, German and Italian)

Tai Chi for Osteoporosis

Tai Chi for Diabetes (available in English and Korean)

Tai Chi for Older Adults

Tai Chi 4 Kidz

Qigong for Health

Tai Chi—the 24 Forms

Tai Chi—the 32 Sword Forms

Intermediate and advanced series are also available.

Dr Paul Lam also has a website: www.taichiproductions.com. It contains tai chi information, discussions, lists of tai chi instructors worldwide, and up-to-date products from Dr Lam's team. Dr Lam's company, Tai Chi Productions, is dedicated to improving people's health and quality of life by promoting Dr Lam's Tai Chi for Health programs through research, education and instructional materials.

Appendix

Enrich your tai chi practice with imagery
by Dr Yanchy Lacska and Dr Paul Lam

Yanchy's personal experience
My first tai chi experience was as a student in a once-per-week community education class in a high school gymnasium. The teacher was Douglas Bowes, a long-time student of T. T. Liang. I remember how much I enjoyed the class and how each week I felt like I was finally learning and memorizing the form—that is, until I got home. Each week I would leave the class excited to practise, only to arrive at home and forget at least some of what we had been taught. It took me several weeks before I came to a realization that I might correct this situation by applying a technique that I had learned and used as a psychologist. I began to apply this technique to help resolve my frustrating dilemma.

This is what I began to do. At the end of each practice, I would walk to my car, sit behind the steering wheel and imagine myself doing the tai chi forms. After mentally going through the forms a few times, I would drive home and then practise the forms physically again.

The technique I was using is known as active imagery. Active imagery is a means to mentally practise, and to communicate to ourself our conscious intent. This is not a new process, even in the West. In the 1970s, professional golfer Jack Nicklaus said that he never hit a shot without first imagining the perfect flight and flawless landing of the ball on the green.

In the late 1980s, I was coaching my daughter's community youth basketball team. I remember an experiment I had the girls carry out during practice. I asked them to execute ten free throws each and count the number of baskets they made. Next I had them sit down, close their eyes, and imagine, in detail, standing at the free throw line and preparing to shoot. I led them step by step through imagery culminating with the ball cleanly swooping through the net. Next I had them shoot ten free throws again. The percentage of baskets successfully completed improved dramatically for each and every girl on the team.

Modern research

Lao Tze says in the Tao te Ching, "Without going outside, you may know the whole world." In a modern scientific equivalent, Harvard neuroscientist, Steven Kosslyn, has demonstrated that when people imagine things, the parts of their brains involved with the senses they are using in their imagining become active. When people imagine moving, for example, the areas of the prefrontal motor cortex that instruct the body to move become active. The brain therefore, cannot easily distinguish between actually doing tai chi forms and imagining doing tai chi forms.

Dr Richard M. Suinn of Colorado State University took the imagery process to a new level with the development of viseo-motor behaviour rehearsal or VMBR. This process combines deep relaxation with vivid mental imagery of the skill to be learned. Researchers at Texas State University used this method in a study of students in a beginners' karate class. The class was divided into two groups. One group received only karate training. The other group was taught VMBR along with the karate instruction. The class met two times per week for six weeks. At the end of the six weeks, students were asked to complete an anxiety inventory before being tested on karate skills. They also used their new skills in sparring. The VMBR group reported less anxiety, scored better on the skills test and scored more points in sparring than the karate-only group.

Dr Kate Lorig works with groups of people who have arthritis at Stanford University. She and her colleagues also teach a combination of relaxation with imagery. Participants imagine performing exercises or skills with their joints loose and pain free. Those who use this combination regularly report less pain and improved physical and psychological functioning. In addition, they make only about half of the doctor visits that they made for their arthritis before using relaxation and imagery.

Using mental imagery in tai chi

The first step in using imagery effectively is relaxation. Lao Tze said, "Empty yourself of everything, return to the source of stillness." This is a good description of relaxation. There are many relaxation techniques you can try. To begin deep relaxation, close your eyes and start to breath using the diaphragm or belly. As you inhale, allow the belly (diaphragm) to naturally expand. As you exhale, draw the belly back in. This is called diaphragmatic or dan tian breathing in qi gong and tai chi practice.

To develop this method, imagine that air travels past your nose to the trachea or the breathing tube, fills up the lungs, and then continues to travel down to fill up the abdomen. As you imagine air travelling to the dan tian, your abdomen swells up; as you imagine it being expelled, your abdomen contracts. Keep the breathing slow, even, and continuous, and in the same tempo as your tai chi movement. Breathing should not be forced. If there is any feeling of discomfort, you should go back to normal breathing.

Next, use the form of abdominal breathing often referred to as "natural breathing". After several breaths, complete a mental body scan, working your way down from the top of your head. Focus on each part of the body and relax any tension you feel in that part of the body each time you exhale. Continue this process until you mentally reach the soles of your feet.

There are many other relaxation methods you can read up on, such as progressive muscle relaxation, systematically tensing and relaxing muscle groups, or autogenic training. Relaxation has benefits besides preparing you for your tai chi imagery work. Regular, deep relaxation can reduce blood pressure and enhance the immune system. Research at the Menninger Clinic in Houston, USA found that people who can achieve a state of deep relaxation often experience insight into problems they are working to resolve. The relaxed state can produce receptive imagery from the unconscious, which helps us to discover our needs and our potential for problem solving.

Time to focus

Once your body is relaxed, your mind is calm and you are no longer thinking about that report due at work or school or what is for dinner, it is time to begin the imagery practice. In order to utilize imagery to the fullest you must first focus your attention on the skill you wish to enhance—in this case, your tai chi. Focus all of your attention on a clear and vivid image of yourself standing ready to begin your tai chi forms. If interfering thoughts or images enter your mind, take a deep breath and allow the images to pass by as you exhale. Then refocus on the tai chi image.

Imagery should not to be confused with visualization. Imagery, in fact, does not require visualization to be effective. The objective in using imagery to enhance tai chi play is not to see pretty pictures in your mind, but to pay attention, to be mindful, to train the body and mind. Imagery can utilize any or all of the senses. It certainly can include visual imagery, but may also include images of sounds, kinaesthetic sensations, and even smells.

I remember attending workshops during which the presenter guided us through a visualization experience for relaxation. I always felt frustrated because I could not see anything with my eyes closed. The leader would be saying in a soft, soothing voice, "You are walking along the beach and now you come to the shore. You see the blue sky and the white sand. The beautiful blue-green water beckons to you." I found myself getting more tense instead of relaxed, thinking, "Hey! I'm not even at the beach yet. Wait for me." It was only later, during my training in clinical hypnosis, that I began to experience imagery through my other senses. I discovered that while I couldn't see the beach, I could feel the warm sun and feel the sand between my toes.

Now that you have achieved a clear image of yourself standing ready to begin your tai chi, you can develop the active imagery. Imagine beginning the commencement form in vivid detail. Use your breath as you would when doing the form physically. Imagine the shifting of your weight and the gentle raising of your arms. Imagine what it feels like to take the first step of your form and how the body moves from the waist. Feel the transfer from substantial to insubstantial. Imagine completing the movements to perfection. Continue this detailed imagery for every form. When you have mentally rehearsed all of the forms, continue for a few minutes with relaxed dan tian breathing, allowing the images to settle and become part of your being. After you have completed your routine mentally, practise it physically. It is interesting to practise the forms before your imagery works and then again after your imagery session and note how the experience changes.

Practical guides

Using imagery during your tai chi practice reinforces that the mind is the master and the body must follow. We would now like to use a movement to illustrate how you can use imagery to enhance your tai chi learning. We have chosen the 24 Forms because it is the best known tai chi set. We will use Movement 7: Stroking the Bird's Tail (left) (see p. 140)

* From the previous move, standing with your weight on the right foot and the ball of the left foot touching the ground, hold your hands as if you were carrying a ball, with the right hand on top. Keep a space between the hands and chest, and keep your body upright and supple.

* Step out to the left with your toes pointing to the left, hands moving very slightly, right hand towards left and left hand towards right, as though you're gently squeezing the ball. This is to initiate the next movement of the hand to the opposite direction.

* Push your left arm forward to form a semicircle in front of your chest and move your right hand next to your hip, with the fingers forward. At the same time, shift your weight forward gradually. Imagine the left arm is pushing gently against an opponent's hand, using the forward shifting of weight to power your left arm.

* Imagine your opponent is now punching you with his or her right fist from your left side. You continue to shift your weight forward slightly and, with a slight turn of the waist, turn your left hand out so that it is resting on your opponent's elbow joint, and the right hand is holding the opponent's fist—you are touching your opponent getting ready to receive this incoming force.

* As your opponent punches forward, you follow his or her force, yield by shifting your weight back and bring both arms down to absorb the incoming force, then you guide the direction of this force by moving your hands to the right.

* Slowly bring both hands up, moving them in a gentle arc.
* Imagine your opponent is retreating since his force has been absorbed and redirected, he or her is losing balance, so to gain his or her balance back the opponent is trying to retreat. Imagine you are following your opponent's movement with your right palm pressing onto your left wrist, shift your weight forward halfway and you are turning back to face the opponent, getting ready to deliver force if necessary.
* As your opponent is continuing to retreat, you follow with your force by using your right hand to push the left arm forward to form a semicircle in front of your chest, and shift your weight forward.
* Now imagine your opponent is using both hands to push you, so you spread your hands out in front of you, palms down so that your hands hold on to the wrists of your opponent.
* As he or she pushes forward, you bring your hands and weight back to absorb the incoming force, keeping your torso upright to maintain good balance.
* As the opponent's force becomes weaker (hasn't been absorbed by you) bring your hands down to redirect his or her hands, and sink the qi to the dan tian getting ready to deliver force.
* As he or she is retreating, you push your hands forward and then upwards in a curve, to push him or her away at the same time pushing upwards to uplift your opponent's sinking down force.

When the mind controls the body, it also means that the mind is calm and has good clarity. Thus, when you are fighting, a clear and calm mind will enable you to make better decision. This solo practice will not only help you to remember your movements, but it will also help you learn how to integrate body, mind and spirit.

Letting go of tai chi

Comment by Sheila Rae, master trainer of the Tai Chi for Health programs from Tennessee, USA.

The very act of letting go implies that we are in possession of a thing. When we apply this concept to tai chi, we understand that without learning and practising the form, we do not possess tai chi awareness. But this awareness is not a product of perfected moves and steps only. While good form is vital to the overall experience, it is not the end goal for the serious practitioner.

There comes a point in our practice where we must learn to let go of the form, the perfectionism, and the ego. As we begin tai chi, the ego is good because it helps us to see what we can achieve. It is powerful, fun, and exciting. But like anything we practise to learn, e.g., piano, dance, even cooking, there comes a time when we must let go of trying to follow the prescribed pattern and let the art move through our souls.

We must ask ourselves what is our purpose in learning tai chi. We learn form to become formless; to integrate mind, body and spirit. We learn the principles of tai chi to become accountable to ourselves, not to judge others, but to teach by example how tai chi extends beyond the physical form. When we can use the principles of tai chi to let go and flow in all our activities, we naturally begin to influence our tai chi practice.

If we constantly train to perfect the moves of tai chi, we can't realise the true bliss of doing tai chi. When we let go of the form, wonderful connections can happen. First the moves connect together effortlessly, and then we can connect to the true essence of blending with our environment, with others, and with the universe itself.

I urge you to release the exactness in order to embrace the wholeness that is tai chi.

Index

Acknowledgements

From Paul Lam

This book took several years to develop and complete, thanks to my co-author Nancy's great enthusiasm and inspiring writings. I would like to thank the thousands of tai chi friends, students and instructors who have helped us with their ideas and support. The tai chi form, the Six Easy Steps for Beginners, on which this book is based, took over 15 years to shape and refine. Many people contributed significantly to its development including Ian Etcell, Julie King, John Mills and Sybil Wong whose knowledge and enthusiasm made this program possible.

I'm especially grateful to the instructors and students of my tai chi school—Better Health Tai Chi Chuan Inc. And to my workshop manager Anna Bennett as well as to my USA director Celia Liu and staff of Tai Chi Productions, I admire and am thankful for your dedication to our tai chi vision and for making it possible for me to spend time on this book. My family has also contributed significantly to this project, thanks to my wife, Eunice, for helping me formulate essential concepts, to my son, Matthew, for lending us his graphic genius, and to my daughter, Andrea, for having the vision to take the cover photograph of me during our holidays in New Zealand.

Both Nancy and I are especially grateful to our publisher Helen Bateman for her dedication to excellence and faith in us. Thank you, too, to her colleague Jayne Denshire, editor Scott Forbes and designer Lena Lowe for all their work. We also thank our friends and colleagues all over the world whose photos have appeared in the book and who have shared their positive energy and spirit with us. And a special thank you to Dr Pam Kircher; Caroline Demoise; Pat Lawson and Jeff Morris, master trainers of the Tai Chi for Health programs, who have read and commented on the manuscript. We are most grateful to Dr Yanchy Lacska and Sheila Rae for permission to use your articles.

From Nancy Kaye

I want to thank my first tai chi teacher, Jan Diepersloot, for starting me on the path to better health and increased enjoyment of life. He also introduced me to the joys of teaching.

And then there's my co-author, Paul Lam, who took me up to another plateau in the world of tai chi and instructing. Paul, thank you for being my teacher, and even more important, one of my dearest, most understanding friends.

Speaking of friends, I must acknowledge all the wonderful people I've met over the years through tai chi. There's something special about most tai chi people… Also, a special mention to my close, lifelong tai chi friends Sally and Earl Flage, Debby Wheeler, Marney Ackerman and Robin Malby. And I can't forget to thank those particular friends whose success stories inspired me in writing this book. They'll know who they are.

Thank you to my partner, Lou Satz, for his love and for his patience while I wrote and rewrote. And to my six children, Doug, Sally, Ellen, Julie, Matt and Leigh, I love you and thank you for being grown up. Otherwise, I couldn't have co-authored this book.